DOT/FAA/AM-01/15

Office of Aerospace Medicine
Washington, DC 20591

Index of International Publications in Aerospace Medicine

Melchor J. Antuñano
Katherine Wade
Civil Aerospace Medical Institute
Federal Aviation Administration
Oklahoma City, OK 73125

August 2001

Final Report

This document is available to the public
through the National Technical Information
Service, Springfield, VA 22161.

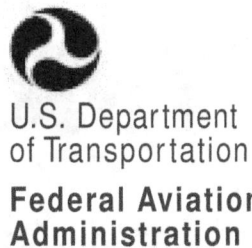

U.S. Department
of Transportation

Federal Aviation Administration

NOTICE

This document is disseminated under the sponsorship of the U.S. Department of Transportation in the interest of information exchange. The United States Government assumes no liability for the contents thereof.

Technical Report Documentation Page

1. Report No. DOT/FAA/AM-01/15	2. Government Accession No.	3. Recipient's Catalog No.
4. Title and Subtitle Index of International Publications in Aerospace Medicine		5. Report Date August 2001
		6. Performing Organization Code
7. Author(s) Antuñano, M.J., and Wade, K.		8. Performing Organization Report No.
9. Performing Organization Name and Address FAA Civil Aerospace Medical Institute P.O. Box 25082 Oklahoma City, OK 73125		10. Work Unit No. (TRAIS)
		11. Contract or Grant No.
12. Sponsoring Agency name and Address Office of Aerospace Medicine Federal Aviation Administration 800 Independence Ave., S.W. Washington, DC 20591		13. Type of Report and Period Covered
		14. Sponsoring Agency Code

15. Supplemental Notes

16. Abstract

The *Index of International Publications in Aerospace Medicine* is a comprehensive listing of international publications in clinical aerospace medicine, operational aerospace medicine, aerospace physiology, environmental medicine/physiology, diving medicine/physiology, aerospace human factors, as well as other topics directly or indirectly related to aerospace medicine. The Index is divided into six major sections: I) Open Publications in General Aerospace Medicine, II) Government Publications in General Aerospace Medicine, III) Publications in Other Topics Related to Aerospace Medicine, IV) Proceedings From Scientific Meetings in Aerospace Medicine and Psychology, V) Journals, Newsletters, and Bulletins in Aerospace Medicine and Aerospace Human Factors, and VI) On-line Databases Containing Bibliographic and Regulatory Information in Aerospace Medicine and Related Disciplines.

17. Key Words Aerospace Medicine, Accident Investigation, Bibliography, Diving, Human Factors, Physiology	18. Distribution Statement Document is available to the public through the National Technical Information Service; Springfield, VA 22161		
19. Security Classif. (of this report) Unclassified	20. Security Classif. (of this page) Unclassified	21. No. of Pages 45	22. Price

Form DOT F 1700.7 (8-72)   Reproduction of completed page authorized

Index of International Publications in Aerospace Medicine

FOREWORD

This manuscript, revised as of July 2001, contains a comprehensive listing of international publications in Clinical Aerospace Medicine, Operational Aerospace Medicine, Aerospace Physiology, Environmental Medicine/Physiology, Diving Medicine/Physiology, Aerospace Human Factors, as well as other important topics directly or indirectly-related to aerospace medicine. This bibliographic guide is divided into six major sections: I) Open Publications in General Aerospace Medicine, II) Government Publications in General Aerospace Medicine, III) Publications in Other Topics Related to Aerospace Medicine and Aerospace Human Factors, IV) Proceedings From Scientific Meetings, Conferences, and Symposiums in Aerospace Medicine and Psychology, V) Journals, Newsletters, and Bulletins in Aerospace Medicine and Aerospace Human Factors, and VI) On-line Computerized Databases Containing Bibliographic Information in Aerospace Medicine and Related Disciplines.

With respect to the type of publications included in this bibliographic guide, our primary objective was to provide the reader with detailed information about "books." Books were selected because they offer a comprehensive coverage of a general area of interest, and they represent excellent tools for structured learning and consultation. On the other hand, article citations from periodical publications (journals, bulletins, and newsletters) were kept to a minimum because their coverage is usually limited to specific issues. Articles are very useful to colleagues who have an adequate understanding of a given general discipline and wish to keep up with the latest developments in the various areas that confirm such a discipline. However, the inclusion of thousands of individual article and technical report citations was beyond the scope of this bibliographic guide. For those colleagues interested in periodical publications, our guide includes a section containing general information on journals, bulletins, and newsletters in Aerospace Medicine and Aerospace Human Factors, indicating which are currently being published on a regular basis and which have been discontinued. Citations to technical reports are included in the numerous indices, bibliographies, serial publications, and on-line databases that are listed throughout the guide.

We believe this guide will be useful as a primary source of consultation for bibliographic information, especially to those colleagues who are in their formative years and to those who do not have easy access to computer-aided literature search systems.

This guide was not intended to be an all-inclusive listing of every publication in aerospace medicine available worldwide. Obviously, there are other publications that we are not aware of due to limitations in our literature search methodologies. Therefore, we take this opportunity to encourage readers to let us know of any publication (old or recent) not listed in this guide that should be included.

Finally, it is important to establish that this bibliographic guide does not constitute a recommendation or an endorsement of any of the publications listed herein. The merits and limitations of each publication should be judged by the reader, keeping in mind that some of these publications should be evaluated as historical documents and not as up-to-date consultation sources.

CONTENTS

I) Open Publications in General Aerospace Medicine --- 1
II) Government Publications in General Aerospace Medicine --- 5
III) Publications in Other Topics Related to Aerospace Medicine --- 6
    Aeromedical Certification and Standards --- 6
    Operational Aerospace Medicine --- 7
    Aeromedical Care and Air Ambulances --- 9
    Aerospace Medicine for Flight Crews --- 10
    Medical Aspects of Aviation Safety and Accidents --- 11
    Aviation and Environmental Physiology --- 13
    Space Physiology, Medicine, and Human Factors --- 17
    Diving Physiology and Medicine --- 24
    Aerospace Human Factors and Psychology --- 27
    General Human Factors and Psychology --- 31
    Aerospace Medicine History --- 33
IV) Proceedings From Scientific Meetings in Aerospace Medicine and Psychology --- 35
V) Journals, Newsletters, and Bulletins in Aerospace Medicine and Aerospace Human Factors --- 37
VI) On-line Databases Containing Bibliographic and Regulatory Information in Aerospace Medicine and Related Disciplines --- 40

Index of International Publications in Aerospace Medicine

I) OPEN PUBLICATIONS IN GENERAL AEROSPACE MEDICINE

Aczél G. A Gyáli Uti Kórház Ünnepi Tudományos Ülésének Elöadásai. Budapest, Hungary: Gyáli Uti Kórház, 1960.

Anderson HG. The Medical and Surgical Aspects of Aviation. London, England: Oxford University Press, 1919.

Anton M. Indreptar de Medicina si Psichologie Aeronautica. Buscuresti, Romania: Editura Military, 1976.

Apollonov AP. Fundamentals of Aviation Medicine. Toronto, Canada: University of Toronto Press, 1943.

Apollonov AP, Voiachek VI. Osnovy Aviatsionnoi Meditsiny. Moskva, USSR: Institut Aviatsionnoi Meditsiny, 1939.

Armstrong HG. Aerospace Medicine. Baltimore, MD, USA: Williams & Wilkins Co., 1961.

Armstrong HG. Principles and Practice of Aviation Medicine. Baltimore, MD, USA: Williams & Wilkins Co., 1939, 1943, 1952.

Artelli M. Legislazione Sanitaria, Marittima e Aeronautica. Milano, Italy: Giuffrè, 1964.

Babiichuk AN. Aviatsionnaia Meditsina. Moskva, USSR: DOSAAF SSSR, 1980.

Baranski S. Medycyna Lotnicza I Kosmiczna. Warszawa, Poland: Panstwowy Zaklad Wydawn, 1977.

Barr EO. Flying Men and Medicine. New York - London: Funk and Wagnalls Co., 1943.

Bauer LH. Aviation Medicine. Baltimore, MD, USA: Williams & Wilkins Co., 1926.

Bauer LH, Christian HA. Aviation Medicine. New York, NY, USA: Oxford University Press, Chap. 14. (Reprinted from Oxford Loose-Leaf Medicine), 1943.

Beier W, Dorner E. Probleme der Raumflugmedizin. Leipzig, Germany: Veb Georg Thieme, 1961.

Benford RJ. Doctors in the Sky. Springfield, IL, USA: Charles C. Thomas, 1955.

Bergin KG. Aviation Medicine - Its Theory and Application. Bristol, England: John Wright & Sons Ltd., 1949.

Bondarenko MR, Braude AI. Voprosy Morfologii, Fiziologii, Biokhimii I Aviatsionnoi Meditsiny. Moskva, USSR: Nauchnye Trudy Tsentral'nogo Ordena Lenina Instituta, 1968.

Boque N. Vida Humana y Espacio. Barcelona, Spain: Jims Editorial Company, 1965.

Box A. Tratado de Medicina Aeronáutica y Aviación. Ceuta, Spain: Impresora Rosaura, 1936.

Boyer J, Strumza MV. Précis d'Hygiene Aéronautique. Paris, France: Expansion Scientifique Française, 1956.

Caidin M, Caidin G. Aviation and Space Medicine - Man Conquers the Vertical Frontier. New York, NY, USA: E. P. Dutton & Co., Inc., 1962.

Chang HY. Hang K'ung Hsin Hsüeh Kuan Ping Chi Ch'u Lin Ch'uang. Pei-ching, China: Jen Min Chün I Ch'u Pan She, 1991.

Ching LP. Hang K'ung I Hsüeh Kai Shu. Taipeh, Taiwan: Chêng Chung Shu Chü, 1955.

Colin J. Médecine Aérospatiale. Paris, France: Expansion Scientifique Publications, 1999.

Covas Coro R. Medicina Aeronáutica: Conferencias de Medicina Aplicada a la Aviación. La Habana, Cuba: Rodriguez, 1949.

Covas Coro RC. Medicina Aeronáutica: Lecciones de Oftalmología, Cardiología, Psicoanálisis y Fisio-Patología en Aviación. La Habana, Cuba: Universidad de la Habana, 1953.

Dal Fabbro G. La Medicina d'Aviazione di Linea. Torino, Italy: Minerva Medica, 1973.

DeHart RL. Fundamentals of Aerospace Medicine. Philadelphia - London: Lea & Febiger, 1985.

DeHart RL. Fundamentals of Aerospace Medicine. Baltimore, MD, USA: Williams & Wilkins, 1996.

Demidov AV. Aviatsionnaia Toksikologiia. Moskva, USSR: Meditsina, 1967.

Dhenin G. Aviation Medicine. Vol. 1: Physiology and Human Factors; Vol. 2: Health and Clinical Aspects. London, England: Tri-Med Books Ltd., 1979.

Diringshofen H. Medizinischer Leitfaden für Fliegende Besatzungen; it Einem Anhang Erste Hilfe bei Flugunfällen. Dresden, Germany: T. Stinkopff, 1939.

Section I. Open Publications in General Aerospace Medicine

Dvorák J, Moravek M. Some Problems of Aviation and Space Medicine. Prague, Czechoslovakia: Charles University, 1967.

Ellingson HV. Medical Problems of Modern Air Travel. Philadelphia, PA, USA: F. A. Davies Co., 1960.

Engle E, Lott AS. Man in Flight - Biomedical Achievements in Aerospace. Annapolis, MD, USA: Leeward Publications, Inc., 1979.

Ernsting J, King P. Aviation Medicine. England - USA: Butterworths, 1988.

Ernsting J, Nicholson, A. Aviation Medicine. England – USA: Butterworth-Heinemann, 1999.

Esteban Aranguez M. Las Funciones Visuales en Aeronáutica. Madrid, Spain: Ediciones Morata, 1941.

Evrard, E. Precis de Medicine Aeronautique et Spatiale. Paris, France: Maloine, 1975.

Fiumel A. Higiena Lotnika: Podrecznik Zbiorowy do uzytku Personelu Latajacego. Warszawa, Poland: Naklad Komitetu Propagandy Medycyny Lotniczej w Polsce, 1937.

Fiumel A, Konopka S. Dziesieciolecie Sluzby Zdrowia w Lotnictwie, 1928-1938. Warszawa, Poland: Instytut Badan Lekarskich Lotnictwa, 1938.

Fulton JF. Aviation Medicine in Its Preventive Aspects. London, England: Oxford University Press, 1948.

Galla E. Repülöorvostan. Budapest, Hungary: Zrinyi Kiadó, 1956.

Gallouin L. Essai de Classification Documentaire de Medicine Aeronautique. Paris, France: Expansion Scientifique Francaise, 1949.

Gerecht K. Biochemische und Physiologische Veranderungen bei Piloten von Segelflugzeugen Wärend Längerer Flüge. Köln, Germany: Deutsche Forschungsanstalt für Luft-und Raumfahrt, 1989.

Giurdzhian AA. Anglo-Russkii Slovar' po Aviatsionno-Kosmicheskoi Meditsine, Psikhologii I Ergonomike. Moskva, Russia, 1997.

Grandpierre R. Elements de Medicine Aeronautique. Paris, France: L'expansion Scientifique Française, 1948.

Grossmann K. Flugmedizin: Leitfaden für die Praxis. Köln, Germany: Deutscher Ärzte-Verlag, 1985.

Guimares G. Compendio de Medicina Aeronautica. Rio D.F., Brazil: Companhia Impresora e Editora Paulista, 1947.

Gurevich II, Medvedev NN. Voprosy Aviatsionnoi Meditsiny. Moskva, USSR: Izd-vo Inostrannoi Lit-ry, 1954.

Hang K'ung I Hsüeh Pien Wei Hui. Hangkong Yixue. Pei-ching, China: Jen Min Chün I Ch'u Pan She, 1992.

Harding RM, Mills J. Aviation Medicine - Articles from the British Medical Journal. London, England: Derry and Sons Ltd., 1983, 1988.

Harding RM, Mills J. Aviation Medicine. London, England: BMJ Publishing Group, 1993.

Hardjoloekita S. Ilmu Kesehatan Penerbangan. Djakarta, Indonesia: Pembangunan, 1955.

Huszcza A. Zarys Wsploczesnej Metodyki Badan Lotniczo-Lekarskich. Warszawa, Polond: Komitet Propagandy Medycyny Lotniczej w Polsce, 1936.

Ikegami H. Hiko to Karada. Tokyo, Japan: Hobun Shorin, 1971.

International Air Transport Association. IATA Medical Manual. Montreal, Canada: IATA Medical Advisory Committee, 1979.

International Civil Aviation Organization. Manual of Civil Aviation Medicine. DOC-8984-AN-895, 2nd Edition. Montreal, Canada: ICAO, 1985.

Isakov PK. Teoriia I Praktika Aviatsionnoi Meditsiny. Moskva, USSR: Meditsina, 1971.

Jokl E. Aviation Medicine. Glendale, England: Arthur C. Clark Publishing Co., 1942.

Jokl E. Medical Aspects of Aviation. London, England: Sir Isaac Pitman & Sons Ltd., 1943.

Jones IH. Flying Vistas: The Human Being, as Seen Through the Eyes of the Flight Surgeon. London - Philadelphia: J. B. Lippincott Co., 1943.

Joy M. First European Workshop in Aviation Cardiology. England – USA: Academic Press, 1992.

Joy M. Second European Workshop in Aviation Cardiology. England – USA: Saunders, 1999.

Kameda H. Koku Igaku to Uchu Igaku. Tokyo, Japan: Fuji Rebio, 1994.

Koku Igaku Jikkentai. Waga Kuni ni Okeru Koku Igaku Bunken Mokuroku. Tokyo, Japan: Koku Igaku Jikkentai, 1963.

Koku Igaku Kenkyu Senta. Kokuki Join no Igaku Tekisei Kenkyu Hokokusho. Tokyo, Japan: Koku Igaku Kenkyu Senta, 1997.

Koku Igaku Kenkyu Senta. Kokuki Join no Karei to Igaku Tekisei Kenkyu. Tokyo, Japan: Koku Igaku Kenkyu Senta, 1990.

Koku Igaku Kenkyu Senta. Rinsho Koku Igaku. Tokyo, Japan: Homeido Shoten, 1995.

Komendantov GL. Voprosy Aviatsionnoi Meditsiny. Moskva, USSR: Trudy Tsentral'nogo Ordena Lenina Instituta Usovershenstvovaniia Vrachei, 1970.

Komendantov GL. Voprosy Aviatsionnoi Meditsiny, Normal'noi I Patologicheskoi Fiziologii. Moskva, USSR: Trudy Tsentral'nogo Instituta Usovershenstvovaniia Vrachei, 1966.

Konopka S. L'Aviation et la Medicine: Bibliographie pour l'Annee 1935. Varsovie, Poland: Edition du Comite de Propagande de Medecine Aeronautique en Pologne, 1937.

Kraft MA. Medical Aspects of Civil Aviation. New York, NY, USA: Flight Safety Foundation, 1958.

Landgraf H. Flugreisemedizin. Germany – USA: Blackwell Wissenschafts-Verlag, 1996.

Lavnikov AA. Aviatsionnaia Meditsina. Moskva, USSR: 1961.

Lavnikov AA. Osnovy Aviatsionnoi Meditsiny. Moskva, USSR: Voennoe Izd-vo Ministerstva Oborny SSSR, 1971.

Lavnikov AA. Principles of Aviation and Space Medicine (translated from the Russian). Washington DC, USA: National Aeronautics and Spce Administration, 1977.

Lomonaco T. L'Assistenza Aero-Medica per il Personale Pilota D'Aeronautica. Rome, Italy: Instituto di Medicina Sociale, 1968.

Lomanaco T. L'uomo in Volo: Manuale di Medicina Aeronautica per il Personale Aeronavigante. Rome, Italy: Abruzzini, 1950.

Lomonaco T, Scano A, Lalli G. Medicina Aeronautica ed Elementi di Medicina Spaziale. Rome, Italy: Regionale Editrice, 1959.

Lovelace WR, Gagge AP. Aviation Medicine and Psychology: A Report Prepared for the AAF Scientific Advisory Group. Wright Field, OH, USA: Headquarters Air Material Command, 1946.

Lubiczkowa J. Test Statokinezjometryczny w Ocenie Stanu Równowagi. Warszawa, Poland: Wojskowego Instytutu Medycyny Lotniczej w Warszawie, 1975.

Malmejac J. Medecine de L'Aviation - Bases Physiologiques et Physio-Pathologiques. Paris, France: Libraries de L'Academie de Medicine, 1948.

Mason JK, Reals WJ. Aerospace Pathology. Chicago, IL, USA: College of American Pathologists Foundation: 1973.

Mayo Aero Medical Unit. Studies in Aviation Medicine. Rochester, MN, USA, 1946.

Menghetti A. Lezioni de Medicina Legale Militare Aeronautica. Firenze, Italy: Scuola de Guerra Aerea, 1960.

Mercier AEG. Visual Problems in Aviation Medicine. New York, NY, USA: Macmillan, 1962.

Milano A. Higiene Militar y del Aviador. Buenos Aires, Argentina: Establecimiento Tipográfico Ferrari Hermanos, 1925.

Monaco A, Gemeli A, Margaria R. Trattato de Medicina Aeronautica. Volumes I, II and III. Rome, Italy: Ufficio Editoriale Aeronautico, 1942.

Moravek M, Dvorak J. Some Problems of Aviation and Space Medicine. Prague, Czechoslovakia: Charles University Press, 1967.

Muller B. Flugmedizin: Kompendium der Luftfhrtmedizin. Dusseldorf, Germany: Droste Verlag, 1956.

Muller B. Flugmedizin - Fur die Arztliche Praxis. Bonn, Germany: Kirschbaum Verlag, 1973.

Nastoiu I. Bazele Metabolice ale Medicinii Aerosptiale: cu Aplicatii în Medicina si Biologie. Bucuresti, Romania: Editura Medicala, 1983.

North Atlantic Treaty Organization – Advisory Group for Aerospace Research and Development. Collected Papers on Aviation Medicine. London, England: Butterworth Scientific Publications, 1955.

North Atlantic Treaty Organization – Advisory Group for Aerospace Research and Development. Neurological, Psychiatric, and Psychological Aspects of Aerospace Medicine. Neuilly-sur-Seine, France: AGARD, 1991.

North Atlantic Treaty Organization – Advisory Group for Aerospace Research and Development – Aerospace Medical Panel. Cardiopulmonary Aspects in Aerospace Medicine. Neuilly-sur-Seine, France: AGARD, 1993.

Novikov VS. Korrektsilia Funktsional'nykh Sostoianii pri Ekstremal'nykh Vozdeistviiakh. Sankt-Peterburg, Russia: Nauka, 1998.

Nyström EV. Flygmedicin: Förste Flygläkare. Stockholm, Sweden: P.A. Norstedt & Söners, 1951.

Papenfuss W. Luftfahrtmedizin: mit Einer Einführung in die Raumfahrtmedizin. Berlin, Germany: Brandenburgisches Verlagshaus, 1990.

Parin V. Aviatsionnaya i Kosmicheskaya Meditsina. Moscow, USSR: Akademiya Meditsinskikh Nauk, 1963.

Parin VV. Kosmicheskaia Kardiologiia. Leningrad, USSR: Meditsina, 1967.

Section I. Open Publications in General Aerospace Medicine

Parin VV, Khazen IM. Aviakosmicheskaia Meditsina. Moskva, USSR: Trudy, 1967.

Pavlok J. Speciální Hygiena Letce. Praha, Czechoslovakia: Státní Zdravotnické Nakl., 1954.

Perrin de Brichambaut, Behaghe P. Trastornos Orgánicos a que están sometidos los Aviadores: sus causas, sus explicaciones y sus remedios. Buenos Aires, Argentina: Imprenta Rinaldi Hermanos, 1924.

Pescador del Hoyo L. Medicina Aeronáutica: el Vuelo de Alta Cota. Barcelona, Spain: Ediciones Científico Médica, 1941.

Piñeiro Sorondo J. Socorro Médico Aéreo en Ortopedia y Traumatología. Buenos Aires, Argentina: Imprenta Sebastián de Amorrotu y Hijos, 1941.

Pintillie I. Studii si Cercetari de Medicina se Psihologie Aeronautica si Spatiala. Bucuresti, Romania: Centrul de Medicina Aeronautica, 1980.

Platonov KK. Chelovek v Polete. Moskva, USSR: 1957.

Puga CR. Manual de Fisiopatología del Hombre en Vuelo. Buenos Aires, Argentina: Instituto Nacional de Medicina Aeronáutica, Talleres Gráficos de Aeronáutica, 1953.

Randel HW. Aerospace Medicine. Baltimore, MD, USA: Williams & Wilkins Co., 1971.

Rayman RB. Clinical Aviation Medicine. New York, NY, USA: Vantage Press, 1982.

Rayman RB. Clinical Aviation Medicine. Philadelphia - London: Lea & Febiger, 1990.

Rayman RB. Clinical Aviation Medicine. New York, NY, USA: Castle Connolly Graduate Medical Publishing, 2000.

Rudnyi NM. Aviatsionnaia Meditsina. Moskva, USSR: Meditsina, 1986.

Ruff S, Strughold H. Atlas der Luftfahrtmedizin. Leipzig, East Germany: Barth, 1942.

Ruff S, Strughold H. Compendium of Aviation Medicine. Leipzig, East Germany: Johan Ambrosius Barth, 1939.

Schick FV. Untersuchung der Pulsfrequenzvariabilität als Schätzgrösse der Pilotenbeanspruchung bei Anthropotechnischen Experimenten. Köln, Germany: Deutsche Forschungs-und Versuchsanstalt für Luft-und Raumfahrt, 1979.

Schmidt I. Bibliographie der Luftfahrtmedizin; eine zusammenstellung von abeiten uber luftfahrtmedizin und grenzgebiete bis ende 1936. Berlin, Germany: J. Springer, 1938.

Schneider J. Luftfahrt - Medizin. Coburg, Germany: Verlag der Weltlfhthart, 1952.

Schnell W. Luftfahrtmedizin; Einführung in die Biologie und Hygiiene des Flugwesens. Berlin, Germany: C.J.E. Volckmann Nachfl, 1935.

Schulze E. Flugmedizin. Berlin, Germany: Transpress, 1990.

Sergeev AA. Otechestvennaia Literature po Aviatsionnoi, Vysokogornoi, I Kosmicheskoi Biologii I Meditsine. Leningrad, USSR: Nauka, 1969.

Soldano HA. Medicina Aeronáutica. San José, Costa Rica: José Loisi Gráficas, 1949.

Strumza MV. Médecine Aérospatiale. Paris, France: Editions Médicales et Universitaires, 1977.

Strumza MV. Médecine Aérospatiale: Certificat d'Études Spéciales de Médicine Aéronautique de l'Unité d'Enseignement et de Recherches Biomédicale. Paris, France: Éditions Médicales Universitaires, 1973.

Sundgren NE. Luftfartsmedicin; Referat och Utdrag. Stockholm, Sweden: Flygvapnet, 1941.

Szczesniak AB. Wojskowy Instytut Medycyny Lotniczij. Warszawa, Poland: Wydawn Ministerstwa Obrony Narodowej, 1988.

Tsai C. Hang K'ung I Hsüeh Ju Mên. Shanghai, China: Hua-Tung I Wu Shêng Huo Shê, 1951.

Tsai C, Feng KC. Hang K'ung Yü K'ung Chien I Hsüeh Chi Ch'u. Pei-ching, China: Kuo Fang Kung Yeh Ch'u Pan She, 1979.

Velasco Diaz DC. Medicina Aeronáutica: Actuaciones y Limitaciones Humanas. Madrid, Spain: Editorial Paraninfo, 1995.

Vlasov VD. Chelovek v Aviatsii i Bezopasnost' Poletov. Moskva, Russia: Assotsiatsiia Aviatsionnoi I Kosmicheskoi Meditsiny Rossii, 1998.

Wang TH. Chung I Yü Hang Ping Hsüeh. His-an, China: Shen-his K'o Hsüeh Chi Shu Ch'u Pan She, 1996.

Werne S. Flygmedicinsk Orientering. Lund, Sweden: Gleerups, 1949.

White CS, Lovelace II WR, Hirsch FG. Aviation Medicine - Selected Reviews. New York, NY, USA: Pergamon Press, 1958.

Whittingham H. Aviation Medicine. London, England: Butterworths, 1950.

II) GOVERNMENT PUBLICATIONS IN GENERAL AEROSPACE MEDICINE

Armée de l'Air. État Major Général. Médecine Aéronautique. Hygiène-Survie. Paris, France: Armée de l'Air, 1966.

Bergeret P. *Aeronautical Preventive Medicine*. Paris, France: North Atlantic Treaty Organization (NATO), Advisory Group for Aeronautical Research and Development, Aerospace Medical Panel, 1957.

Birley JL. Medical Problems of Flying. Special Report Series No. 53. London, England: Medical Research Council, His Majesty's Stationery Office, 1920.

Centro de Investigación de Medicina Aeronáutica. Ciencias Astronáuticas y Medicina Espacial. Madrid, Spain: Gráficas Virgen de Loreto, 1966.

Centro di Studi e Ricerche di Medicina Aeronautica. Raccolta Pubblicazioni Scientifiche: 1938-1950. Guidonia, Italy: Centro di Studi e Ricerche di Medicina Aeronautica, 1951.

Collins WE, Wayda ME. Index of FAA Office of Aviation Medicine Reports: 1961 through 2000. DOT/FAA/AM-01/1. Oklahoma City, OK, USA: Federal Aviation Administration, Civil Aeromedical Institute, 2001.

Crowley JS, Bruckart J. United States Army Aviation Medicine Handbook. Fort Rucker, AL, USA: Society of U.S. Army Flight Surgeons, 1993.

Garcia Conde M, Gallego LC. Primer Ciclo de Conferencias de Ciencias Astronáuticas y Medicina Espacial. Madrid, Spain: Centro Instrucción Medicina Aeroespacial, 1965.

Jones GM. DRB Aviation Medical Research Unit Reports. Ottawa, Canada: Defense Research Board, 1971.

Kafka MM. Flying Health. Harrisburg, PA, USA: Military Service Publishing Co., 1942.

Kerr WK. Bibliography of Canadian Reports in Aviation Medicine: 1939-1945. DR-153. Canada: Defense Research Board, Department of National Defense, 1962.

Kornaszewski W. Higiena Lotnicza Wydawnictwo. Warszawa, Poland: Ministerstwa Obrony Narodowej, 1958.

Lomonaco T. Elementi di Fisiologia e Patologia dell' uomo in Volo. Roma, Italy: Ministero dell' Aeronautica, Stabilimento Fotomeccanico, 1946.

Lomonaco T. L'uomo in Volo. Roma, Italy: Ministero dell' Aeronautica, Stabilimento Fotomeccanico, 1950.

Lopez Coterilla V. Medicina Aeronáutica y Espacial. Madrid, Spain: Centro Instrucción Medicina Aeroespacial, 1968.

Ministerio de Sanidad y Seguridad Social. Salud y Aviación Civil. Madrid, Spain: Instituto de Estudios de Sanidad y Seguridad Social, 1981.

Naval Aerospace Medical Institute. U.S. Naval Flight Surgeon's Manual. Washington, DC, USA: Office of Naval Research, Bureau of Medicine and Surgery, U.S. Department of the Navy, 1978.

Naval Aerospace Medical Institute. United States Naval Flight Surgeon's Manual. Virtual Naval Hospital, USA: 2000.

North Atlantic Treaty Organization. A Glossary of Terms Commonly Used in Aviation Medicine. London, England: NATO Advisory Group for Aeronautical Research and Development, Aerospace Medical Panel, 1959.

Office of Director of Air Service. Aviation Medicine in the Army Expeditionary Force. Washington, DC, USA: U. S. Government Printing Office, 1920.

Platonow K. Der Menschim Fluge. Berlin, Germany: Ministeriums for Nationale Verteidigung, Verlag Des., 1959.

Rayman RB, USAF Air War College, Air University. Aviation Medicine - Its Clinical Applications. USAF-FR-270-32-0881. Washington, DC, USA: U.S. Government Printing Ofice, 1977.

Robinette JC. Bibliography on Aeromedical Research with Abstracts. Dayton, OH, USA: USAF Aerospace Medical Research Laboratory, Wright-Patterson Air Force Base, Wright Air Development Division, 1960.

School of Aviation Medicine. Flight Surgeon's Handbook. San Antonio, TX, USA: Randolph Field, Army Air Forces, 1943.

Society of USAF Flight Surgeons. Flight Surgeons Check List. San Antonio, TX, USA: USAF School of Aerospace Medicine, 1984.

Society of USAF Flight Surgeons. Flight Surgeons Check List. San Antonio, TX, USA: USAF School of Aerospace Medicine, 1993.

U.S. Air Force Surgeon General. German Aviation Medicine - World War II. Volumes I and II. Washington, DC, USA: U.S. Government Printing Office, 1950.

Section II. Government Publications in General Aerospace Medicine

U.S. Army. Army Flight Surgeons Manual. ST-71-22. Fort Rucker, AL, USA: U.S. Army Aeromedical Center, 1976.

U.S. Army. Medical Research Laboratory. Manual of Medical Aspects of Aviation. [] USA: U.S. Army, 1918.

U.S. Bureau of Medicine and Surgery. Aviation Medicine Practice. Pensacola FL, USA: School of Aviation Medicine and Research, Naval Air Station, 1955.

U.S. Congress. House. Committee on Transportation and Infrastructure. Subcommittee on Aviation. Pilot Fatigue: Hearings before the Subcommittee on Aviation of the Committee on Transportation and Infrastructure, One Hundred Sixth Congress, First Session, August 3 and September 15. Washington, DC, USA: U.S. Government Printing Office, 2000.

U.S. Department of the Air Force. Flight Surgeon's Manual. AFM-160-5. Washington, DC, USA:1954.

U.S. Department of the Air Force. Flight Surgeon's Manual. AFM-161-1. Washington, DC, USA: 1962.

U.S. Department of the Navy. Naval Flight Surgeons Manual. Washington, DC, USA: U.S. Government Printing Office, 1978.

U.S. National Library of Medicine. Bibliography of Space Medicine. Washington, DC, USA: National Library of Medicine, Reference Division, 1958.

U.S. Navy School of Aviation Medicine and Research, Aviation Medicine Division, Bureau of Medicine and Surgery. Aviation Medicine Practice. Washington, D C, USA: Bureau of Naval Personnel, 1955.

U.S. War Department. Air Service Medical Manual. Washington, DC, USA: U.S. Government Printing Office, 1919.

U.S. War Department. Notes on Cardiology in Aviation Medicine. Washington, DC, USA: U.S. Government Printing Office, 1940.

U.S. War Department. Notes on Eye, Ear, Nose, and Throat in Aviation Medicine. Washington, DC, USA: U.S. Government Printing Office, 1940.

U.S. War Department. Notes on Physiology in Aviation Medicine. Washington, DC, USA: U.S. Government Printing Office, 1940.

Wilmer WH. Aviation Medicine in the A. E. F. Washington, DC, USA: U.S. Government Printing Office, War Department, 1920.

III) PUBLICATIONS IN OTHER TOPICS RELATED TO AEROSPACE MEDICINE

Aeromedical Certification and Standards

Association Médicale Canadienne. Le Médecin et la Loi sur l'Aéronautique: Guide sur la Déclaration Obligatoire. Ottawa, Canada: Association Médicale Canadienne, 1995.

British Air Ministry. The Medical Examination of Civilian Aviators. London, England: C.A. Pub. # 1, 1928.

Canadian Medical Association. Fit for Flying? A Guide for Mandatory Medical Reporting. Canada, 1985.

Civil Aviation Authority. The Avoidance of Fatigue in Aircrews: Guide to Requirements. Cheltenham, England: 1994.

Civil Aviation Authority. Guidance Notes for Authorized Aviation Medical Examiners. London, England: 1986.

Davis FB. The AAF Qualifying Examination. Washington, DC, USA: U.S. Government Printing Office, 1947.

DeHaan WV. The Optometrist's and Ophthalmologist's Guide to Pilot's Vision: A Practical Guidebook for Dealing with all Clinical Aspects of Pilot's Vision Requirements. USA: American Trend Publishing Co., 1982.

Dickson ED. Contributions to Aviation Otolaryngology. London, England: Headly Brothers, 1947.

Federal Aviation Administration. Aeromedical Certification Statistical Handbook. Oklahoma City, OK, USA: Civil Aeromedical Institute, 1998.

Federal Aviation Administration. Guide for Aviation Medical Examiners. Washington, DC, USA: Office of Aviation Medicine, 1999.

Fries IB. The Pilot's Medical Advisor: A Guide to Obtaining and Keeping Your Medical Certificate. Greenwich, CT, USA: Belvoir Publications, 1995.

International Civil Aviation Organization. International Standards and Recommended Practices - Personnel Licensing. Annex 1 to the Convention on International Civil Aviation, 8th Edition. Montreal, Canada, 1988.

Krol J. Medical Examination and Standards: Medical Requirements, Waivers and Restrictions for Aircrew. Soesterberg, Netherlands: Netherlands Aerospace Medical Centre, 1998.

Lovelace Foundation for Medical Education and Research. Seminar for Aviation Medical Examiners. Albuquerque, NM, USA: Lovelace Foundation, 1962.

Maublanc, R. Medical Examination of Airmen. New York, NY, USA: William Wood and Co., 1921.

Maublanc PA, Ratié VC. Guide Practique pour l'Examen Médical des Aviateurs, des Candidate à l'Aviation et des Pilotes. Paris, France: J.B. Baillière et Fils, 1920.

Pérez Sastre JM, Guillen Gallego PY. Guia Práctica para Médicos Examinadores Aéreos. Madrid, Spain: Ministerio de Transportes, 1985.

Perry CJG. Psychiatry in Aerospace Medicine. Boston, MA, USA: Little Brown Co., 1967.

Reinhart RO. FAA Medical Certification: Guidelines for Pilots. Ames, IA, USA: Iowa State University Press, 1997.

Royal Air Force - Air Ministry. Manual for Medical and Dental Officers of the Royal Air Force. London, England: His Majesty's Stationery Office, 1940.

Royal Air Force - Air Ministry. The Medical Examination for Fitness for Flying. London, England: His Majesty's Stationery Office, 1936.

Sutherland GA. The Examination of Aviation Candidates. Lancet, 1918, II:803.

U.S. Department of the Air Force. Medical Examination and Medical Standards. Air Force Regulation 160-43. Washington, DC, USA: Headquarters USAF, 1983.

U.S. War Department – Surgeon General. Notes on Psychology and Personality Studies in Aviation Medicine. Washington, DC, USA: U.S. Government Printing Office, 1941.

U.S. War Department - Surgeon General. Outline of Neuropsychiatry in Aviation Medicine. Washington, DC, USA: U.S. Government Printing Office, 1940.

Operational Aerospace Medicine

Aerospace Medical Association, Air Transport Medicine Committee. Medical Guidelines for Airline Travel. Alexandria, VA, USA: Aerospace Medical Association, 1997.

Aerospace Medical Association, Committee on Aviation Toxicology. Aviation Toxicology. New York, NY, USA: Blakiston Co., 1953.

Agrelo RAM. Notas de Higiene Aeronautica: Apuntes sobre Directivas para Pasajeros de los Aviones de Transporte. Buenos Aires, Argentina: 1947.

Anderson EG. The Pilot's Health. Blue Ridge Summit, PA, USA: Tab Books, 1984.

Association Nationale des Anciens Parachutistes. Pathologie du Parachutisme. Paris, France: Maloine, 1984.

Bada Ainsa JL, Foz Tena A. Normas Sanitarias para Viajeros a Países Tropicales: Atlas Médico de las Enfermedades Tropicales. Barcelona, Spain: Universitat Automona de Barcelona, 1993.

Bailey J. Guide to Hygiene and Sanitation in Aviation. Geneva, Switzerland: World Health Organization, 1977.

Barish RJ. The Invisible Passenger: Radiation Risks for People Who Fly. Madison, WI: Advanced Medical Publishing, 1996.

Billings CE, Ashe WF. The Medical Aspects of Business Aviation. Columbus, OH, USA: Ohio State University Press, 1962.

Bond DD. How Can the Flight Surgeon Better Treat Anxiety ? New York, NY, USA: Josiah Macy Jr. Foundation, 1945.

Bond DC. The Love and Fear of Flying. New York, NY, USA: International Universities Press Inc., 1952.

Chapman P. Airline Medical Manual. London – USA: Chapman and Hall Medical, 1991.

Cook DL. Vision: What Every Pilot Needs to Know. Atlanta, GA, USA: Invision Press, 1991.

Corachán Cuyás M, Genové M. Salud y Viajes. Manual de Consejos Práticos. Barcelona, Spain: Ediciones Científicas y Técnicas, 1993.

Cruchet R, Mouliner R. Air Sickness. New York, NY, USA: William Wood and Co., 1920.

Curtis T. Understanding Aviation Safety Data: Using the Internet and Other Sources to Analyze Air Travel Risk. Warrendale, PA, USA: Society of Automotive Engineers, 2000.

Cutting WC. Guide to Drug Hazards in Aviation Medicine. Washington, DC, USA: Federal Aviation Administration - Aviation Medical Service, U.S. Government Printing Office, 1962.

Dawood R. Traveller's Health. Oxford, England: Oxford University Press, 1986.

Dearnaley EJ, Warr PB. Aircrew Stress in Wartime Operations. London, England: Academic Press, 1979.

Dix MR, Hood JD. Vertigo. Chichester, England: J. Wiley & Sons, 1984.

DuPont HL, Steffen R. Textbook of Travel Medicine and Health. Canada – USA: Blackwell Science, 1997.

Section III. Publications in Other Topics Related to Aerospace Medicine

Esteban Aranguez M. Las Funciones Visuales en Aeronáutica. Madrid, Spain: Editorial Morata, 1941.

Fabbro GD. La Medicina D'Aviazione di Linea. Rome, Italy: Edizioni Minerva Medica, 1973.

Forgione AG, Bauer FM. Fearless Flying. Boston, MA, USA: Houghton Mifflin Co., 1980.

Greist JH, Greist GL. Fearless Flying - A Passenger Guide to Modern Airline Travel. Chicago, IL, USA: Nelson-Hall, 1981.

Henderson VE. Air Crew in their Element: Hints for the Maintenance of Fitness and Confidence. Toronto, Canada: University of Toronto Press, 1942.

Her Majesty's Stationery Office. The Public Health (Aircraft) Regulations. London, England: HMSO, 1979

Herrero Aldama P, Santandreu L. Aspectos de la Fatiga de Vuelo. Madrid, Spain: CIMA, 1978.

Herrero Aldama P, Santandreu L. Bajas por Enfermedad e Incapacitació en Aviación. Madrid, Spain: SEPLA/IBERIA, 1977.

Holbrook HA. Civil Aviation Medicine in the Bureaucracy. Bethesda, MD, USA: Banner Publishing Co., 1974.

International Civil Aviation Organization. Manual on Prevention of Problematic Use of Substances in the Aviation Workplace. Montreal, Quebec, Canada: International Civil Aviation Organization, 1995.

Kahn FS. The Curse of Icarus: The Health Factor in Air Travel. England – USA: Routledge, 1990.

Koku I, Kenkyu S. Kokuki Join on Igaku Tekisei Kenkyu Hokokusho. Tokyo, Japan: Heisei, 1993.

Leduc JF. Notions de Médecine Aéronautique à l'Usage des Infirmières d'Aviation Sanitaire et du Personnel Navigant de l'Aéronautique. Paris, France: 1936.

Leimann-Patt HO, Moia PI. Factores Psicosomáticos que Incrementan la Susceptibilidad a la Cinetosis. INMAE-PC-87-09. Buenos Aires, Argentina: Instituto Nacional de Medicina Aeronáutica y Espacial, 1987.

Leimann-Patt HO, Moia PI. Síndromes de Desadaptación Secundaria al Vuelo. Buenos Aires, Argentina: Sociedad Interamericana de Psicología Aeronáutica, 1989.

Leitmann P. Sindromes de Desadaptación Secundaria al Vuelo. Buenos Aires, Argentina: Sociedad Interamericana de Psicologia Aeronáutica, 1989.

Marquis R. Hygiène Pratique de l'Aviateur et de l'Aéronaute. Paris, France: A. Malione, 1912.

McFarland RA. Fatigue in Aircraft Pilots. New York, NY, USA: Philosophical Library, 1942.

Ministerio de Sanidad y Consumo. La Salud También Viaja. Consejos y Normas Sanitarias para Viajeros Internacionales. Madrid, Spain: Ministerio de Sanidad, 1990.

Nagda NL. Air Quality and Comfort in Airliner Cabins. West Conshohocken, PA, USA: ASTM, 2000.

National Academy of Sciences - National Research Council. Night Visibility. Washington, DC, USA: U.S. Government Printing Office, 1958.

National Academy of Sciences, National Research Council. The Role of Fatigue in Pilot Performance. Washington, DC, USA: NRC Committee on Selection and Training of Aircraft Pilots, U.S. Government Printing Office, 1946.

National Research Council, Committee on the Effects of Aircraft-Pilot Coupling on Flight Safety. Aviation Safety and Pilot Control: Understanding and Preventing Unfavorable Pilot-Vehicle Interactions. Washington, DC: National Academy Press, 1997.

North Atlantic Treaty Organization - Advisory Group for Aerospace Research and Development - Aerospace Medical Panel. Selection and Training Advances in Aviation. Neuilly-sur-Seine, France: AGARD, 1996.

Office of the Chief of Naval Operations. Night Vision for Airmen. Washington, DC, USA: U.S. Government Printing Office, 1944.

Parliament, House of Lords – Select Committee on Science. Air Travel and Health. London, England: Stationery Office, 2000.

Pérez Sastre JM. Conceptos Básicos de Medicina y Psicología Aeronáutica para Pilotos. Madrid, Spain: American Flyers España, 1994.

Plat C. Secourisme Aeronautique. Paray-Vieille-Poste, France: Institut de Formation Aeronautique, 1993.

Prieto Zancudo C. Guia del Viajero. Madrid, Spain: INSALUD, 1993.

Reason JT, Brand JJ. Motion Sickness. New York, NY, USA: Academic Press, 1975.

Reinhart RO. Fit for Flight: Flight Physiology and Human Factors for Aircrew. Ames, IA, USA: Iowa State University Press, 1999.

Reitz G, Schnuer K. Radiation Exposure of Civil Aircrew. Ashford, Kent, England: Nuclear Technology Publishing, 1993.

Ribak J, Rayman RB. Occupational Health in Aviation: Maintenance and Support Personnel. San Diego, CA, USA: Academic Press, 1995.

Sarnoff CA. Medical Aspects of Flying Motivation. Brooks AFB, San Antonio, TX, USA: USAF School of Aerospace Medicine, 1957.

Schröetter HR. Hygiene der Aëronautik. Leipzig, Germany: Grethlein & Company, 1909.

Schröetter HR. Hygiene der Aëronautik und Aviatik. Vienna – East Germany: Wilhelm Braumüller, 1912.

Skjenna OW. *Cause Factor: Human.* ???, Canada. Minister of National Health and Welfare, 1981.

Smith GM, Dismukes K. Facilitation and Debriefing in Aviation Training and Operations. England – USA: Ashgate, 2000.

Smith PW, U.S. Department of Transportation, Federal Aviation Administration. Medical Problems in Aerial Application. Washington, DC, USA: U.S. Government Printing Office, 1977.

Stellungnahme der Strahlenschutzkommission. Die Ermittlung der Durch Kosmiche Strahlung Verursachten Strahlenexposition des Fliegenden Personals. Germany – USA: Gustav Fischer, 1995.

Stevens R, Luciani, R. Plane Truth: Tips for Combating the Health and Safety Perils of Flying. Far Hills, NJ, USA: New Horizon Press, 1994.

Thom T. The Air Pilot's Manual: Vol. 6. Human Factors and Pilot Performance. Shrewsbury, England: Airlife, 1997.

Ursano RJ, Holloway HC. Aerospace Operations. In Kaplan HI and Sadock BJ. Comprehensive Textbook of Psychiatry. Baltimore - London: Williams and Wilkins Co., 1985.

Vaandrager K, Ide HC. Consideraciones Médicas en la Aviación Comercial. Caracas, Venezuela: KLM Royal Dutch Airlines, 1960.

Wright DG. Notes on Men and Groups under Stress of Combat for the Use of Flight Surgeons in Operational Units. New York, NY, USA: Josiah Macy Jr. Foundation, 1945.

Aeromedical Care and Air Ambulances

Bare WW. How to Choose An Air Ambulance That's Safe. Blackwood, NJ, USA: ANAAA, 1990.

Bare WW. Medical Care in the Air - A Training Manual for the Aeromedical Attendant. Blackwood, NJ, USA: ANAAA, 1990.

Bare WW. Protect Your Patient in the Air! Air Ambulance Standards for the Association of North American Air Ambulances. Blackwood, NJ, USA: ANAAA, 1982.

Campbell DN. Wings of Mercy: A Living History of Saskatchewan's Air Ambulance Service, North Battleford, Saskatchewan, Canada: Turner-Warwick Publications, 1993.

Dorland P, Nanney J. Dust off: Army Aeromedical Evacuation in Vietnam. Washington, DC, USA: U.S. Army Center of Military History, 1982.

Genell L. Flight Nursing. National Flight Nurse Association. Saint Louis, MO, USA: Mosby-Year Book, 1990.

Grant JS. Medical Services in Transport. London, England: Butterworth, 1966.

Health and Welfare Department of Canada, Medical Services Branch. Patient Care in Flight: Manual for Medical Services Personnel. Canada: Medical Services Branch, 1985.

Holleran RS. Flight Nursing: Principles and Practice. St. Louis, MO, USA: Mosby, 1997.

Holleran RS. Mosby's Emergency and Flight Nursing Review. St Louis, MO, USA: Mosby, 1996.

IBERIA Dirección Servicios al Cliente. Pasajeros con Movilidad Reducida. Consejos para el Viaje. Madrid, Spain: IBERIA, 1990.

Lam DM. Aeromedical Evacuation: A Handbook for Physicians. San Antonio, Texas, USA: USAF School of Aerospace Medicine, Brooks AFB, 1980.

Lee G. Flight Nursing: Principles and Practice. St. Louis, MO, USA: Mosby-Year Book, 1991.

Martin T. Aeromedical Transportation: A Clinical Guide. Brookfield, VT, USA: Avebury Aviation, 1996.

Maycock R. 1957. Doctors in the Air. London, England: G. Allen & Unwin Publishing Co., 1957.

McNeil EL. Airborne Care of the Ill and Injured. New York, NY, USA: Springer-Verlag, 1983.

Ministère de la Guerre, Direction du Service de Santé. Les Avions Sanitaires: Leur Évolution, Leur Emploi. Paris, France: G. Roche d'Estrez, 1923.

Ministerio del Aire. Transporte de Pasajeros Enfermos. Madrid, Spain: Ministerio del Aire, Servicio Información Aeronáutica, 1956.

National Air Transportation Association. NATA Bloodborne Pathogens Exposure Rule Guidelines for Air Ambulance Operators. Alexandria, VA, USA: National Air Transportation Association, 1994.

Section III. Publications in Other Topics Related to Aerospace Medicine

National Highway Traffic Safety Administration and the American Medical Association Commission on Emergency Medical Services. Air Ambulance Guidelines. Washington, DC, USA: U.S. Department of Transportation. 1981.

Orr P. Manual for Aeromedical Evacuation. Canada: Northern Medical Unit, University of Manitoba Press, 1984.

Pérez Sastre JM, Moreno Milán E. Manual Sanitario para Tripulantes de Cabina de Pasajeros. Madrid, Spain: Arán Ediciones, 1999.

Salinas JC, Ruiz Boada F. I Jornadas Civico-Militares de Sanidad. Madrid, Spain: Sanidad y Consumo, 1985.

Samuels D, Bock H. Air Medical Crew National Standard Curriculum: Advanced Student Manual. Pasadena, CA, USA: ASHBEAMS, 1988.

Solivellas M. Iniciación al Aerotransporte Sanitario y en Ambulancias Asistidas. Palma de Mallorca, Spain: Gobierno de Baleares, 1986.

Sredl DM. Airborne Patient Care Management: A Multidisciplinary Approach. St. Louis, MO, USA: Medical Research Associates Publications, 1983.

Task Force on Interhospital Transport. Guidelines for Air and Ground Transport of Neonatal and Pediatric Patients. Elk Grove Village, IL, USA: American Academy of Pediatrics, 1999.

Tracy JP, Norcross JA. Doc Flighty. Fallbrook, CA, USA: Aero Publishers, 1965.

U.S. Department of the Air Force - Office of the Surgeon General. Concise History of the United States Air Force Aeromedical Evacuation System. Washington, DC., U.S.A: U.S. Government Printing Office, 1976-626-850-379.

U.S. National Highway Traffic Safety Administration. Air Ambulance Guidelines. Washington, DC, USA: U.S. Department of Transportation, 1986.

Aerospace Medicine for Flight Crews

Brown HN. Pilot's Aeromedical Guide. Blue Ridge Summit, USA: TAB Books, 1980.

Caudevilla P, Ortiz P. Conceptos Básicos de Medicina y Psiología Aeronáutica para Pilotos. Madrid, Spain: American Flyer, 1996.

Cruchet R, Moulinier R. Le Mal des Aviateurs, ses Causes et ses Remédes. Paris, France: J.B. Balliére et Fils, 1920.

Diringshofen HV. Medical Guide for Flying Personnel. Toronto, Canada: University of Toronto Press.

Ferry G. L'Aptitude à l'Aviation, le Vol en Hauteur et le Mal des Aviateurs. Paris, France: J.B. Ballière et Fils, 1918.

Ferry G. Influence du Vol en Avion sur la Santé de l'Aviateur. Nancy, France: Berger-Levrault, 1920.

Grow MC, Armstrong HG. Fit to Fly. A Medical Handbook for Fliers. London, England: D. Appleton-Century Company, 1942.

Hansen WB. Fit to Fly: An Aeromedicine Handbook for Pilots. New York, NY, USA: Van Nostrand Reinhold, 1982.

Health and Welfare Canada. The Pilot's Guide to Medical Human Factors. Ottawa, Canada: Canada Communication Group, 1993.

Lomonaco T. Un Medico fra gli Aviatori. Roma, Italy: Regionale Editrice, 1980.

Medical Study Group of BALPA. Fit to Fly - A Medical Handbook for Pilots. London: Granada, 1980.

Mohler SR. Medication and Flying - A Pilot's Guide. Boston, MA, USA: Boston Publishing Company, 1982.

Naval School of Aviation Medicine. Aviation Medicine Technicians' Manual. Pensacola, FL, USA: U.S. Naval Air Station, School of Aviation Medicine, 1993.

Negre Colmillo A, Vila Bennasar JB. Manual de Asistencia Médica Primaria y Educación en Medicina Aeronáutica. Mallorca, Spain: SPANTAX, 1984.

Perrin de Brichambaut P. Critères de l'Aptitude au Vol en Avion. Paris, France: L. Arnette, 1921.

Read KEE. Aeromedicine for Aviators. London, England: Pitman, 1971.

Reinhart RO. The Pilot's Manual of Medical Certification and Health Maintenance. USA: Specialty Press, 1982.

Rosario Saavedra A. Aeronáutica para Pilotos. Madrid, Spain: Sumaas, S.A., 1983.

Tomas Rubio S, Blanes Espi A. Actuaciones y Limitaciones Humanas en Aviación Civil. Valencia, Spain: Tadiar, 1991.

U.S. Army Air Forces. Your Body in Flight: An Illustrated "Book of Knowledge" for the Flyer. Fairfield, OH, USA: Air Service Command, 1943.

U.S. Department of the Air Force. Your Body in Flight. Washington, DC, USA: U. S. Department of the Air Force, 1960.

U.S. Department of the Army. Aeromedical Training for Flight Personnel. Washington, DC, USA: U.S. Army Field Manual ARMY-FM-301, 1979.

U.S. Department of Transportation, Federal Aviation Administration. Medical Handbook for Pilots. Washington, DC, USA: U.S. Government Printing Office, 1974.

Yules RB. The Pilot's Complete Medical Guide. New York, NY, USA: J. Aronson Publishing Co., 1983.

Medical Aspects of Aviation Safety and Accidents

Advisory Group for Aerospace Research & Development. The Prevention of Aircraft Accidents through the Collection and Analysis of Human Factors/Aeromedical Aircraft Accident Data. Neuilly-sur-Seine, France: AGARD, 1998.

Alkov RA. Aviation Safety—the Human Factor: A Handbook for Flight Safety Officers and Aviation Accident Investigators. Casper, WY, USA: Endeavor Books, 1997.

Armed Forces Institute of Pathology, Division of Aerospace Pathology. Aerospace Pathology for the Flight Surgeon. Washington, DC, USA: U.S. Printing Office, 1986.

Barter S. A Rapid Mapping and Analysis System for Use During Aircraft Accident or Incident Field Investigation. Melbourne, Australia: Aeronautical and Maritime Research Lab, 1999.

Beaty D. The Human Factor in Aircraft Accidents. New York, NY, USA: Stein and Day, 1969.

Bergeret PM. Aircraft Accident Investigation Manual for Air Surgeons (NATO). England – USA: Pergamon, 1961.

Bergeret PM. Escape and Survival - Clinical and Biological Problems in Aero Space Medicine. New York - Oxford - London- Paris, Pergamon Press, 1961.

Civil Aeronautics Board. Accidents in Aerial Application Activities. Washington, DC, USA: Bureau of Safety, 1959.

Condon-Rall ME. Disaster on Green Ramp: The Army's Response. Washington, DC, USA: Government Printing Office, 1996.

Coombs C. Survival in the Sky. USA: William Morrow and Co., 1956.

Cushing S. Fatal Words: Communication Clashes and Aircraft Crashes. Chicago, IL, USA: University of Chicago Press, 1997.

Daniel and Florence Guggenheim Aviation Safety Center at Cornell University. Survey of Research Projects in the Field of Aviation Safety: 1951, 1953-1956, 1958-1967. New York, NY, USA: Cornell University Press, 1968.

Dionne G, Gagné R. A Statistical Analysis of Airline Accidents in Canada: 1976-1987. Montreal, Canada: Centre de Recherche sur les Transports, 1992.

Edwards A. Flights into Oblivion. Mclean, VA, USA: Paladwr Press, 1993.

Evrard E, Bergeret P, van Wulfften PM. Medical Aspects of Flight Safety. New York - London - Paris - Los Angeles: Pergamon Press, 1959.

Hasbrook AH. Gross Pattern of Injury of 109 Survivors of Five Transport Accidents. Phoenix, AZ, USA: Cornell University Press, 1958.

Hasbrook AH, Petry RM. Handbook for Aircraft Accident Investigators Cooperating in Crash Injury Research. Ithaca, NY, USA: Cornell University Medical College, 1951.

Hengi BI, Krauthauser J. Crash: Flugzeugunfalle 1945-Heute. Allershausen, Germany: NARA-Verlag, 1993.

Hoekstra HD, Huang SC. Safety in General Aviation. Arlington, VA, USA: Flight Safety Foundation, 1971.

IBERIA. Dirección Técnica de Vuelo. Manual Básico de Operaciones de Vuelo. Madrid, Spain: IBERIA, 1992.

IBERIA. Dirección Técnica de Vuelo. Manual de Seguridad y Salvamento. Madrid, Spain: IBERIA, 1992.

International Air Transport Association. Handling of Human Remains. Airport Handling Manual 353, Section 3, Sheet 1, 1982.

International Civil Aviation Organization. Accident/Incident Reporting Manual, 2nd Edition. Montreal, Quebec, Canada: International Civil Aviation Organization, 1987.

International Civil Aviation Organization. Aircraft Accident and Incident Investigation: International Standards and Recommended Practices: Annex 13 to the Convention on International Civil Aviation, 8th Edition. Montreal, Quebec, Canada: International Civil Aviation Organization, 1994.

International Civil Aviation Organization. Aircraft Accident and Incident Investigation, Part I: Organization and Planning. Montreal, Quebec, Canada: International Civil Aviation Organization, 2000.

International Civil Aviation Organization. Manual of Aircraft Accident Investigation. Montreal, Canada: ICAO 1959.

Section III. Publications in Other Topics Related to Aerospace Medicine

Internationale Bergrettungsärzte-Tagung. Der Internistische Notfall im Gebirge; Die Unfallproblematik Mit Fluggeräten im Alpinen Luftraum. Innsbruck, Austria: Eigenverlag G. Flora, 1993.

Jordanoff A. Safety in Flight. New York, NY, USA: Funk and Wagnalls Co., 1941.

Kawakita T. Tsuiraku Jiko No Ato. Tokyo, Japan: Bungei Shunju, 1992.

Kepert JL. Aircraft Accident Investigation at ARL: The First 50 Years. Fishermens Bend, Victoria, Australia: Aeronautical Research laboratory, 1993.

Koku Igaku Jikkentai. Kokujko ni Kansuru Koku Igaku Bunken Mokuroku. Tokyo, Japan: 1965.

Kowalsky NB. An Analysis of Pilot Error-Related Aircraft Accidents. Albuquerque, NM, USA: Lovelace Foundation, 1973.

Krause SS. Aircraft Safety: Accident Investigations, Analyses, and Applications. New York, NY, USA: McGraw-Hill, 1996.

Mason JK. Aviation Accident Pathology: A Study of Fatalities. London, England: Butterworths & Co. Ltd., 1962.

McCormick BW, Papadakis MP. Aircraft Accident Reconstruction and Litigation. Tucson, AZ, USA: Lawyers & Judges Publishing Company, 1996.

McKinney WJ. Accident Aftermath: A Commander's Handbook. Maxwell AFB, AL, USA: Air University Research Coordinator Office, 1997.

North Atlantic Treaty Organization – Advisory Group for Aerospace Research and Development – Aerospace Medicine Panel. Aircraft Accidents: Trends in Aerospace Medical Investigation Techniques. Neuilly-sur-Seine, France: AGARD, 1992.

North Atlantic Treaty Organization – Advisory Group for Aerospace Research and Development – Aerospace Medicine Panel. Injury Prevention in Aircraft Crashes: Investigative Techniques and Applications. Neuilly-sur-Seine, France: AGARD, 1998.

O'Donell JA., Grimaldi JV. Ground Safety in Aviation Operations. American Museum of Safety and the Center for Safety Education, New York, NY, USA: New York University Press, 1954.

Oster DV, Strong JS. Why Airplanes Crash: Aviaton Safety in a Changing World. New York, NY, USA: Oxford University Press, 1992.

Owen D. Air Accident Investigation: How Science is Making Flying Safer. England – USA: Naynes North America, 1998.

Panas J. Aircraft Mishap Photography: Documenting the Evidence. Ames, IA, USA: Iowa State University Press, 1996.

Reals WJ. Medical Investigation of Aviation Accidents. Chicago, IL, USA: College of American Pathologists, 1968

Ríos-Tejada F. Manual para la Investigación Médica de Accidentes Aéreos. Madrid, Spain: Ministerio de Defensa, 1999.

Royal Canadian Air Force. Down But Not Out. Ottawa, Canada: Queen's Printer, 1965.

Santina HD. Manual of Aviation Pathology. SCHAVMED P-19, Pensacola, FL, USA: U.S. Navy School of Aviation Medicine, 1962.

Sarsfield L. Safety in the Skies: Personnel and Parties in the NTSB Aviation Accident Investigations. Santa Monica, CA, USA: Rand, 2001.

Society of United States Air Force Flight Surgeons. Aircraft Mishap Investigation Handbook. Brooks AFB, TX, USA: Society of USAF Flight Surgeons, 1994.

Society of United States Naval Flight Surgeons. Pocket Reference to Aircraft Mishap Investigation. NAS Pensacola, FL, USA: The Society of U.S. Naval Flight Surgeons, 1995.

Stevens PJ. Fatal Civil Aircraft Accidents. Bristol, England: John Wright, 1970.

Stevens PJ. Fatal Civil Aircraft Accidents - Their Medical and Pathological Investigation. Baltimore, MD, USA: Williams & Wilkins Co., 1970.

Tripartite International Labour Organization. Occupational Health and Safety in Civil Aviation. Geneva, Italy: International Labour Organization, 1977.

U.S. Armed Forces Institute of Pathology, Joint Committee on Aviation Pathology. An Autopsy Guide for Aircraft Accident Fatalities. Washington, DC, USA, 1957.

U.S. Department of the Air Force. Participation in a Military or Civil Aircraft Accident Safety Investigation: Safety. Washington, DC, USA: U.S. Government Printing Office, 1997.

U.S. Department of the Army. Army Accident Investigation and Reporting. Washington, DC, USA: U.S. Government Printing Office, 1994.

U.S. Department of Transportation, Federal Aviation Administration. Aircraft Accident and Incident Notification, Investigation, and Reporting. Washington, DC, USA: U.S. Government Printing Office, 1994.

U.S. Department of Transportation, Federal Aviation Administration. Aircraft Accident Investigation Manual. Washington, DC, USA: U.S. Government Printing Office, 1985.

U.S. National Safety Council. Aviation Ground Operation Safety Handbook. Chicago, IL, USA: National Safety Council, 1977.

U.S. National Transportation Safety Board. Aviation Accident Investigation Symposium, March 1994, Tysons Corner, Virginia. Springfield, VA, USA: National Technical Information Service, 1994.

U.S. National Transportation Safety Board. Investigator's Manual. Washington, DC, USA: National Transportation Safety Board, 1995.

U.S. Office of Naval Operations. Aviation Medical Safety Training Manual. Washington, DC, USA, 1961.

Walters JM, Sumwalt RL. Aircraft Accident Analysis: Final Reports. New York, NY, USA: McGraw-Hill, 2000.

Warren ND. Studies of Aircraft Accident Causation Utilizing the Index of Accident Exposure. Washginton, DC, USA: Human Factors Operations Research Laboratories, 1954.

Watson TW. Unhappy Landings: Why Airplanes Crash. Melbourne, FL, USA: Harbor City Press, 1992.

Wood RH. Aircraft Accident Investigation. Casper, WY, USA: Endeavor Books, 1995.

Zakhar'iants UZ. Psikhofiziologicheskie I Meditsinskie Problemy Bezopasnosti Poletov: mezhvuzovskii Tematicheskii Sbornik Nauchnykh Trudov. Leningrad, USSR: Akademiia Grazhdanskoi Aviatsii, 1989.

Aviation and Environmental Physiology

Acosta J. Historia Natural y Moral de las Indias. Seville, 1590. (English Translation. Natural and Moral History of the Indias. London, England: Blount and Ashley, 1604).

Ackles KN, Macella CM. Bibliography of the Human Protective Systems Division. Ottawa, Canada: Defence and Civil Institute of Environmental Medicine, 1995.

Adolph EF. Physiology of Man in the Desert. New York, NY, USA: Interscience Publishers, 1947.

Airlines War Training Institute. Survival: A Manual for Aircraft Crews Forced Down in all Parts of the World – Including Hints on Living off the Land, Building Shelters, Traveling, Protection Against Disease. Washington, DC, USA: Airlines War Training Institute, 1943.

Alpers BJ. Vertigo and Dizziness. New York, NY, USA: Grune & Stratton, 1958.

Asociación Chilena de Seguridad – Laboratorio de Fisiología del Trabajo. Simposio de Salud Ocupacional en Faenas a Gran Altitud. Santiago, Chile: Asociación Chilena de Securidad, 1995.

Auerbach PS. Wilderness Medicine: Management of Wilderness and Environmental Emergencies. St. Louis, MO, USA: 1995.

Autor AP. Pathology of Oxygen. New York, NY, USA: Academic Press, 1982.

Barbour AB, Whittingham HE. Human Problems of Supersonic and Hypersonic Flight. Oxford - New York: Pergamon Press, 1962.

Battestini Pons R, Vanrell R. El Mal de Montaña. Barcelona, Spain, 1963.

Beaupeurt JE. Ten Years of Human Vibration Research. Wichita, KS, USA: Boeing Company, 1969.

Beaupeurt JE, Chaney RE. Tracking Performance During Whole-Body Vibration. Wichita, KS, USA: Boeing Company, 1964.

Beaupeurt JE, Chaney RE. Visual-Motor Performance during Whole-Body Vibration. Wichita, KS, USA: Boeing Company, 1964.

Beaupeurt JE, Parks DL. Visual Performance Under Whole-Body Vibration. Wichita, KS, USA: Boeing Company, 1963.

Bergeret P. Bio-Assay Techniques for Human Centrifuges and Physiological Effects of Acceleration. New York, NY, USA: Pergamon Press, 1961.

Bert P. La Pression Barométrique, Recherches de Physiologie Expérimentale. Paris, France: Massonet Cie, 1878. (English translation by M. A. Hitchcock and F.A. Hitchcock, Barometric Pressure. Columbus, OH., USA: College Book Co., 1943)

Bhattacharjya B. Mountain Sickness. Bristol, England: John Wright, 1974.

Billings CE, Foley ME, Huie CR. Physiological Effects of Induced Hypoxia During Instrument Flying. Columbus, OH, USA: Ohio State University Press, 1963.

Blockly WV, Hanifan DT. An Analysis of the Oxygen Protection at Flight Altitudes Between 40,000 and 50,000 Feet. Arlington, VA, USA: Psychological Research Associates, 1961.

Section III. Publications in Other Topics Related to Aerospace Medicine

Boothby WM. Respiratory Physiology in Aviation. San Antonio, TX, USA: USAF School of Aviation Medicine, Randolph Field, 1954.

Brendel W, Zink RA. High Altitude Physiology and Medicine. New York, NY, USA: Springer-Verlag, 1982.

Bunning E. Die Physiologische Uhr. Berlin, Germany: Springer Verlag, 1958.

Cabezas PG. Hipoacusias del Aviator. New York, NY, USA: American Institute of Aeronautics and Astronautics, 1972.

Caparo AC. Pathology at High Altitude. Lima, Peru: Universidad de San Marcos Press, 1966.

Ch'iu WY. Kao Hsing Neng Chan Chi G li Hun mi Chih Wei Hsien Yü Fang Fan. T'aipei Shih, Taiwan: I Hsüan t'u Shu Ch'u Pan She, 1997.

Clark C. Acceleration and Body Distortion. Baltimore, MD, USA: Martin Marietta Corp., 1961.

Clark RP, Edholm OG. Man and His Thermal Environment. London, England: Arnold, 1985.

Clementi J. Sur Quelques Effets Physiopathologiques de la Navigation Aérienne: Déductions Pratiques. Paris, France: Jouve & Cie, 1935.

Clerc R. Les Principes de l'Education Physique et Sportive de l'Aviateur: Essai de Mise en Pratique. Nancy, France: Imprimerie Georges Thomas, 1946.

Colquhoun WP. Biological Rhythms and Human Performance. London - New York: Academic Press, 1971.

Corbett C, Bazett H. A Study of the Reaction of Pilots and Observers to Diminished Oxygen Pressure: The Medical Problem of Flying. London, England: British Privy Council, Medical Research Council. Special Report Series No. 53:18-69, 1920.

Coriolis G. Traite de Mechanique des Corps Solides et du Calcul de l'effet des Machines. Paris, France: 1846 (German by C.H. Schnuse, Braunschweig. 1946).

Cornell Aeronautical Laboratory. Manned Supersonic Flight: A Reference Manual. Port Washington, NY, USA: Department of the Navy, 1950.

Croce LM. Elementi di Fisiologia e Patologia Dell'Uomo in Volo. Rome, Italy: Abruzzini Editore,1948.

Cruchet R, Earp JR, Moulinier R. Le Mal des Aviateurs - Air Sickness: Its Nature and Treatment. London, England: J. Bale, Sons & Danielsson Ltd, 1920.

Del Vecchio RJ. Psycho-Physiological Aspects of Flight Safety. Commack, NY, USA: Rodel Press, 1990.

Dmitriev AS. Lavirintnye I Ekstralabirintnye Mekhanizmy Nekotorykh Somaticheskikh I Vegetativnykh Reaktsii no Uskorenie. Minsk, USSR: Nauka I Tekhnika, 1969.

Dupuis H, Zerlett G. The Effects of Whole-Body Vibration. Berlin, Germany: Springer-Verlag, 1986.

Edholm OG. Man - Hot and Cold. London, England: Arnold, 1978.

Edholm OG, Bacharach AL. The Physiology of Human Survival. London - New York: Academic Press, 1965.

Evrard E. Physiologie du Vol: Hygiene de L'Aviateur. Bruxelles, Belgium: Office de Publicite, S.A., 1956.

Fanger PO. Thermal Comfort. New York, NY, USA: McGraw-Hill, 1972.

Faubert D, Cooper BC. Tolerance and Performance Under Severe Transverse (±Gx) Vibration. Baltimore, MD, USA: Martin Company, 1963.

Fitzpatrick FL, Stiles KA. The Biology of Flight. New York, NY, USA: The Macmillan Co., 1942.

Folinsbee LJ, Wagner JA, Borgia JF, Drinkwater BL, Gilner JA, Bedi JF. Environmental Stress: Individual Human Adaptations. New York, NY, USA: Academic Press, 1978.

Folk GE. Textbook of Environmental Physiology. 1st Edition, Philadelphia, PA, USA: Lea & Febiger, 1966.

Folk GE. Textbook of Environmental Physiology. 2nd Edition, Philadelphia, PA, USA: Lea & Febiger, 1974.

Folkard S, Monk TH. Hours of Work. Chichester, England: John Wiley & Sons, 1985.

Fregly AR. Handbook of Sensory Physiology. Berlin, Germany: Springer-Verlag, 1974.

Fregly MJ, Blatteis CM. Environmental Physiology. New York, NY, USA: Oxford University Press, 1996.

Frisancho-Piñeda D, Frisancho-Velarde O. Tratado de Medicina de la Altura. Puño, Peru: Universidad Nacional del Altiplano, 1993.

Gauer OH, Zuidema GD. Gravitational Stress in Aerospace Medicine. Boston, MA, USA: Little Brown Co., 1961.

Gemmill CL. Physiology in Aviation. Illinois - Maryland, USA: Charles C. Thomas, 1943.

Gillies JS. A Textbook of Aviation Physiology. Oxford, England: Pergamon Press, 1965.

Glasser O. Medical Physics III. Chicago, IL, U.S.A.: YearBook Medical Publishers, Inc., 1960.

Grinker RR, Spiegel JP. Men Under Stress. New York, NY, USA: McGraw-Hill Book Co., 1945.

Guglielminetti E. Le Mal des Altitudes: le Mal de Montagne Comparé au Mal de Ballon. Paris, France: Aux Bureaux du Progrès Medical, 1901.

Guyton AC. Aviation, Space, and Deep Sea Diving Physiology. In: Human Physiology and Mechanisms of Disease, Philadelphia, PA, USA: W.B. Saunders, 1992, pages 319-328.

Guyton AC. Aviation, Space, and Deep Sea Diving Physiology. In: Textbook of Medical Physiology, Philadelphia - London - Toronto: W.B. Saunders Company, 1981, pages 541-551.

Guyton AC, Hall JE. Aviation, Space and Deep-Sea Diving Physiology. In: Textbook of Medical Physiology, Philadelphia, PA, USA: W.B. Saunders, 2000, pages 496-509.

Haber H. The Physical Environment of the Flyer. San Antonio, TX, USA: Air University, USAF School of Aerospace Medicine, 1954.

Harris CM, Crede CE. Shock and Vibration Handbook. New York, NY, USA: Mc-Graw-Hill Book Co., 1976.

Hashimoto K, Kogi K. Methodology in Human Fatigue Assessment. London, England: Taylor & Francis, 1971.

Haymes EM, Wells CL. Environment and Human Performance. USA - Canada: Human Kinetics Publishers, Inc. 1986.

Heath D, Williams DR. High-Altitude Medicine and Pathology. England – USA: Oxford University Press, 1995.

Heath D, Williams DR. Man at High Altitude: The Pathophysiology of Acclimatization and Adaptation. Scotland – USA: Churchill Livingstone, 1981.

Held R, Liebowitz HW, Teuber HL. Handbook of Sensory Physiology. Vol. 8. Berlin, Germany: Springer-Verlag, 1978.

Henderson D. Effects of Noise on Hearing. New York, NY, USA: Raven Press, 1976.

Herlitzca A. Fisiologia de Aviazione. Bologna, Italy: N. Zanichelli, 1923.

Hiatt EP. Reports on Human Acceleration. Washington, DC, USA: National Academy of Sciences, 1961.

Hiernaux J. Man in the Heat, High Altitude, and Society. Springfield, IL, USA: C.C. Thomas, 1982.

Howard IP, Templeton WB. Human Spatial Orientation. New York, NY, USA: Wiley, 1966.

Howard IP. Human Visual Orientation. Chichester, England: J. Wiley & Sons, 1982.

Hultgren HN. High Altitude Medicine. Stanford, CA, USA: Hultgren Publications, 1997.

Jayle GE. Night Vision. Springfield, IL, USA: Charles C. Thomas, 1959.

Jedeka LW. Physiological Considerations in Aviation. Burbank, CA, USA: Lockheed Aircraft Corporation, 1942.

Johnson LC, Tepas DI, Colquhoun WP, Colligan MJ. Biological Rhythms, Sleep and Shift Work. New York, NY, USA: Spectrum, 1981.

Jokel E, Blount SG. Exercise and Altitude. Switzerland – USA: Karger, 1968.

Jones IH. Equilibrium and Vertigo. Philadelphia, PA, USA: J.B. Lippincott Co., 1918.

Jongblood J, Noyons AK. Onderzoekingen Gedaan in Het Physiologisch Laboratorium der Rijks-Universiteit te Utrecht. Utrecht, The Netherlands: University of Utrecht, 1932.

Keatinge WR. Survival in Cold Water. Oxford, England: Blackwell Scientific Publications, 1969.

Kornhuber HH. Handbook of Sensory Physiology. Vol. 6, Berlin, Germany: Springer-Verlag, 1974.

Kryter KD. The Effects of Noise on Man. New York, NY, U.S.A: Academic Press, 1970.

Laszczynska J. Termowizyjne Zobrazowania Zmian Efektorowych Ukladu Termoregulacji w Odpowiedzi na Bodziec Niedotlenienia Wysokosciowego: Rozprawa Habilitacjna. Warszawa, Poland: Wojskowy Instytut Medycny Lotniczej, 1998.

Leithead CS, Lind AR. Heat Stress and Heat Disorders. London, England: Churchill, 1964.

León-Velarde F. Hipoxia: Investigaciones Básicas y Clínicas: Homenaje á Carlos Monge Cassinelli. Lima, Peru: IFEA Instituto Francés de Estudios Andiños, 1993.

León-Velarde F, Arregui A. Desadaptación a la Vida en la Grandes Alturas. Lima, Peru: IFEA Instituto Francés de Estudios Andiños, 1994.

Lippert S. Vibration Research. New York, NY, U.S.A: Pergamon Press, 1963.

Luce GG. Body Time. New York, NY, USA: Pantheon Books, 1971.

Lumb AB. Nunn's Applied Respiratory Physiology. England – USA: Butterworth-Heinemann, 2000.

Section III. Publications in Other Topics Related to Aerospace Medicine

McFarland RA. The Effects of Oxygen Deprivation on the Human Organism. U.S. Civil Aeronautics Authority, Tech. Devel. Rep. # 11, Washington, DC, USA: U.S. Government Printing Office, 1941.

McFarland RA. Altitude and the Airman. Pan American Airways Inc., 1938.

McFarland RA, Holway AH. Studies of Visual Fatigue. Boston, MA, USA: Harvard Graduate School of Business Administration, 1942.

Mekjavic IB, Banister EW, Morrison JB. Environmental Ergonomics: Sustaining Human Performance in Harsh Environments. Philadelphia - New York - London: Taylor & Francis, 1988.

Miller RD. Effects of Noise on People. Washington, DC, USA: U.S. Environmental Protection Agency, 1971.

Moore-Ede M, Sulzman F, Fuller C. The Clocks that Time Us. Cambridge, MA, USA: Harvard University Press, 1982.

National Research Council – Working Group on Night Vision. Night Vision: Current Research and Future Directions. Washington DC, USA: National Academy Press, 1987.

National Research Council – Subcommittee on Oxygen and Anoxia. Handbook of Respiratory Data in Aviation: Prepared for the Committee on Medical Research. Washington DC, USA: 1944.

Pandolf KB, Sawka MN, Gonzalez RR. Human Performance Physiology and Environmental Medicine at Terrestrial Extremes. Indianapolis, USA: Benchmark Press, Inc., 1988.

Pollard AJ, Murdoch DR. The High Altitude Medicine Handbook. England – USA: Radcliffe Medical Press, 1998.

Porter R, Knight J. High Altitude Physiology: Cardiac and Respiratory Effects. London, England: Churchill Linvingstone, 1971.

Puglisi-Allegra S, Oiverio A. Psychobiology of Stress. Holland – USA: Kluwer Academic Publishers, 1990.

Reinhart, RO. Basic Flight Physiology. Blue Ridge Summit, PA, USA: TAB Books, 1992.

Reinhart, RO. Basic Flight Physiology. New York, NY, USA: McGraw-Hill, 1996.

Rivolier J. High Altitude Deterioration. New York, NY, USA: S. Karger Publishers, Inc., 1985.

Roach RC. Bibliography of High Altitude Medicine and Physiology. Albuquerque, NM, USA: R. Roach, 1995.

Robinette JC. A Selected Bibliography Concerning Physiological Factors in Aero-Medical Research and Development. Wright-Patterson Air Force Base, OH, USA: 1957.

Rodahl K. The Physiology of Work. England – USA: Taylor & Francis, 1989.

Roget FF. Altitude and Health. London, England: Constable Publishing Co., 1919.

Romero de Tehada y Picatoste M, Suevos Orduña LF. Manual de Fisiología Aeronáutica: Nociones de Equipos de Soporte de Vida, Paracaidismo, Supervivencia y Primeros Auxilios. Valladolid, Spain: Quirón, 1994.

Romero de Tejada M. Manual de Fisiología Aeronáutica. Madrid, Spain: IBERIA. Dirección de Vuelo, 1994.

Rosado Bartolome A. La Enferedad Descompresiva en las Actividades Aeroespaciales. Madrid, Spain: IBERIA, 1994.

Ruff S, Strughold H. Grundriss der Luftfahrtmedizin. München, Germany: J.A. Barth, 1957.

Scano A. Tecnica Fisiologica Aeronautica. Firenze, Italy: Scuola de Guerra Aerea, 1960.

Schubert G. Physiologie des Menschen im Flugzeug. Berlin, Germany: Springer - Verlag, 1935.

Shiraki K, Yousef MK. Man in Stressful Environments: Thermal and Work Physiology. Springfield, IL, USA: C.C. Thomas, 1987.

Simonson E. Physiology of Work Capacity and Fatigue. Springfield, IL, USA: Thomas, 1971.

Slonim NB. Environmental Physiology. Saint Louis, MO, USA: The C. V. Mosby Company, 1974.

Soubies J. Physiologie de L'Aeronaute. Paris, France: G. Steinheil, 1907.

Stanley Aviation Corporation. A Study of the Dynamic Model Technique in the Analysis of Human Tolerance to Acceleration. Washington, DC, USA: National Technical Information Center, 1965.

Starkov PM. The Problem of Acute Hypothermia (translated from the Russian). England – USA: Pergamon Press, 1960.

Šulc J. Letcká Fyziologie. Praha, Czechoslovakia: Naše Vojsko, 1980.

Sundstroem ES. Studies on Adaptation of Man to High Altitudes. Berkeley, CA, USA: University of California Press, 1919.

Sutton JR, Coates G. Hypoxia and Mountain Medicine. Burlington, VT, USA: Queen City Printers, 1992.

Sutton JR, Houston CS. Hypoxia and Molecular Medicine. Burlington, VT, USA: Queen City Printers, 1993.

Sutton JR, Houston CS. Hypoxia, Exercise, and Altitude: Proceedings of the Third Banff International Hypoxia Symposium. New York, NY, USA: A.R. Liss, 1983.

Sutton JR, Houston CS. Hypoxia: The Tolerable Limits. Indianapolis, IN, USA: Benchmark Press, 1988.

Sutton JR, Jones NL, Houston CS. Hypoxia, Man at Altitude. New York, NY, USA: Thieme-Stratton, 1982.

Teichner WH. The Psychophysiology of Thermal Regulation. Amherst, MA, USA: University of Massachusetts, 1963.

Tempest W. Infrasound and Low Frequency Vibration. London, England: Academic Press, 1977.

U.S. Air Force. The Physiological Aspects of Aviation. Philadelphia, PA, USA: Medical Field Service School, Carlisle Barracks, 1933.

U.S. Air Force. Physiology of Flight: Human Factors in the Operation of Military Aircraft. Dayton, OH, USA: Aero Medical Research Laboratory, Wright Field, 1942.

U.S. Department of the Air Force. Physiology of Flight. Washington, DC, USA: U.S. Government Printing Office, 1961.

U.S. Department of Transportation. Physiological Training Manual. Washington, DC, USA: Federal Aviation Administration 1984.

U.S. War Department. Physiological Aspects of Flying and Maintenance of Physical Fitness. Washington, DC, USA: U.S. Government Printing Office, Technical Manual No. 1-705, 1941.

Ursin H, Baade E. Psychobiology of Stress: A Study of Coping Men. New York, NY: Academic Press, 1978.

Van Liere EJ, Stickney JC. Hypoxia. Chicago, IL, USA: University of Chicago Press, 1963.

Vogel JHK. Hypoxia, High Altitude and the Heart. Switzerland – USA: Krager, 1970.

Von Beckh HA. Fisiología de Vuelo. Velocidad. Aceleraciones. Gravitación, Accidentes. Paracaidismo. Cinetosis. Astronáutica. Buenos Aires, Argentina: Editorial Alfa, 1955.

Ward M. Mountain Medicine - A Clinical Study of Cold and High Altitude. London, England: Crosby Lockward Staples, 1975.

Ward M, Milledge JS. High Altitude Medicine and Physiology. London, England: Arnold, 2000.

Weihe WH. The Physiological Effects of High Altitude. Oxford, England: Pergamon Press, 1964.

West JB. High Altitude Physiology. New York, NY, USA: Academic Press, 1981.

West JB, Lahiri SK. High Altitude and Man. Bethesda, MD, USA: American Physiological Society, Clinical Physiology Series, 1984.

Wever R. The Circadian System of Man. New York, NY, USA: Springer-Verlag, 1979.

White S, Benson Jr OO. Physics and Medicine of the Upper Atmosphere. Albuquerque, NM, USA: The University of New Mexico Press, 1952.

Whiteside TDC. The Problems of Vision in Flight at High Altitude. London, England: Butterworth Scientific Publications, 1957.

William KG. The New Frontier - Man's Survival in the Sky. Springfield, IL, USA: Charles C. Thomas, 1959.

Yousef MK, Horvath SM, Bullard RW. Physiological Adaptations - Desert and Mountain. New York, NY, USA: Academic Press, 1972.

Zim HS. Man in the Air - The effects of Flying on the Human Body. New York, NY, USA: Harcourt Brace & Co., 1943.

Space Physiology, Medicine, and Human Factors

Akhutin EA, Giurdzhian AA. Mediko-Biologicheskie Problemy Kosmicheskikh Poletov. Moskva, USSR: Nauka, 1972.

Armstrong HG, Haber H, Strughold H. Aeromedical Problems of Space Travel. J. Aviation. Med., 1949; 20:383-417.

Aroesty J, Zimmerman R. Human Support Issues and Systems for the Space Exploration Initiative: Results from Project Outreach. Santa Monica, CA, USA: Rand, 1991.

Asashima M, Malacinski GM. Fundamentals of Space Biology. Japan – Germany – USA: Springer-Verlag, 1990.

Ashford D, Collins P. Your Spaceflight Manual: How You Could be a Tourist in Space Within Twenty Years. New York, NY, USA: Crescent Books, 1991.

Atkov O, Bednenko VS. Hypokinesia and Weightlessness: Clinical and Physiologic Aspects (translated from the Russian). Madison, CT, USA: International Universities Press, 1992.

Section III. Publications in Other Topics Related to Aerospace Medicine

Austrian Society for Aerospace Medicine. Health from Space Research: Austrian Accomplishments. Austria – USA: Springer-Verlag, 1992.

Baker CA. Visual Capabilities in the Space Environment. New York, NY, USA: Pergamon Press, 1965.

Benson OO, Strughold H. Physics and Medicine of the Atmosphere and Space. New York, NY, USA: John Wiley & Sons Inc., 1960.

Beregovofi GT. Eksperimental'no-Psikhologicheskie Issledovaniia v Aviatsii I Kosmonavtike. Moskva, USSR: Akademiaa Nauk SSSR, 1978.

Berry CA. Space Medicine. JAMA, 1967; 201:232-241.

Berry CA. Space Medicine in Perspective - A Critical Review of the Manned Space Program. JAMA, 1967; 201:232-241.

Berry CA. The Medical Legacy of Gemini - Life Sciences and Space Research. Amsterdam, Holland: North Holland Publishing Co., 1968.

Bio-Dynamics, Inc. Study of the Transferral of Space Technology to Biomedicine. Cambridge, MA, USA: Bio-Dynamics, Inc., 1964.

Bourne GH. Medical and Biological Problems of Space Flight. New York, NY, USA: Academic Press, 1963.

Brown JH. Physiology of Man in Space. New York, NY, USA: Academic Press, 1963.

Brown JL. Sensory and Perceptual Problems Related to Space Flight. Washington, DC, USA: National Academy of Sciences, 1961.

Burns NM. Physiological Problems of Man in Space. New York, NY, USA: Free Press of Glencoe, 1963.

Busby DE. Space Clinical Medicine. Amsterdam, Holland: D. Reidel Publishing Co., 1968.

Calvin M, Gazenko OG. Foundations of Space Biology and Medicine. Vol. I-Space as a Habitat, Vol. II-Ecological and Physiological Bases of Space Biology and Medicine, Vol. III-Space Medicine and Biotechnology. Washington, DC,: U.S. Government Printing Office, NASA Special Publication # 374, 1975.

Campbell PA. Medical and Biological Aspects of the Energies of Space. New York, NY, USA: Columbia University Press,1961.

Caprara G. Living in Space: from Science Fiction to the International Space Station. Canada – USA: Firefly Books, 2000.

Catalano GB, Fortunato V. Relazioni: I Barotraumatimi in O.R.L. e I Loro Aspetti Particolari in Medicina Aeronautica e Spaziale: XVII Conventus, Societas Oto-Rhino-Laringologica Latina. Catania, Italy: Tip dell'Università, 1968.

Centre d'Essais en Vol. Laboratoire Médico-Physiologique. Paris, France: Aviaplans, 1963.

Centre National d'Etudes Spatiale. Physiologie Spatiale. Toulouse, France: Cepadues Editions, 1983.

Churchill SE. Fundamentals of Space Life Sciences. Malabar, FL, USA: Krieger Publishing Company, 1997.

Colin J, Houdas Y. Physiologie du Cosmonaute. Paris, France: Presses Universitaires de France, 1965.

Connors MM, Harrison AA, Akins FR. Living Aloft: Human Requirements for Extended Space Flight. NASA Special Publication # 483, Washington, DC,: U.S. Government Printing Office, 1985.

Denisov VG, Onishchenko VF. Inzhinernaia psikhologiia v Aviatsii I Kosmonavtike. Moskva, USSR: Mashinostroenie, 1972.

Dickson KJ. Space Human Factors Publications, 1980-1990. Washington, DC, USA: National Aeronautics and Space Administration, 1991.

Eckart P. Spaceflight Life Support and Biospherics. The Netherlands – USA: Kluwer Academic, 1996.

Engle E, Lott AS. Man in Flight, Biomedical Achievements in Aerospace. USA: Leeward Publications Inc., 1979.

Flaherty BE. Psychophysiological Aspects of Space Flight. New York, NY, USA: Columbia University Press, 1961.

Fraser TM. Human Responses to Sustained Acceleration. NASA Special Publication # 103. Washington, DC,: U.S. Government Printing Office.

Freeman M. Challenges of Human Space Exploration. England – USA: Springer, 2000.

Frontiers Symposium. The 12th Frontiers Symposium: Pharmacology Beyond Earth's Boundaries. Philadelphia, PA, USA: Lippincott, 1994.

Gagarin Y, Lebedew V. Survival in Space. New York, NY, USA: Frederick A. Praeger, 1969.

Gaisser TK. Cosmic Rays and Particle Physics. England – USA: Cambridge University Press, 1990.

Gantz KF. Man in Space, The United States Air Force Program for Developing the Spacecraft Crew. New York, NY, USA: Duell, Sloan and Pearce, 1959.

Gazenko OG. Kosmicheskaia Biologiia I Meditsina: Sovmestnoe Rossiisko-Amerikanskoe Izdanie v Piati Tomakh. Moskva, Russia: Nauka; Washington D.C., USA: Amerikanskii in-t Aeronavtiki I Astronavtiki, 1994.

George Washington University Medical Center. Crew Interaction in Situations Simulating Long-Term Space Flight. Descriptive Analyses of the Literature. Washington, DC, USA: George Washington University, 1974.

Gerathewohl ST. Principles of Bioastronautics. Englewood Cliffs, NJ, USA: Prentice-Hall, 1963.

Giurdzhian AA, Khvatkov NM. Anglo-Russkii Slovar' po Aviatsionno-Kosmicheskoi Meditsine, Psikhologii i Ergonomike: Okolo 25 000 Terminov. Moskva, Russia: 1997.

Glaister DH. The Effects of Gravity and Acceleration on the Lung. London, England: Technical Press, 1970.

Golovanov AK. Arkhitektura Nevesomosti: Priglashenie k Razmysheniiu. Moskva, Russia: Mashinostroenie, 1985.

Gurevich II, Ivanov VI. Chelovek v Usloviiakh Vysotnogo I Kosmicheskogo Poleta. Moskva, USSR: 1960.

Gurovskii NN. Ocherki Psikhofiziologii Truda Kosmonatov. Moskva, USSR: Meditsina, 1967.

Haber H. Man in Space. 1st Edition, Indianapolis, USA: Bobbs-Merrill, 1953.

Hagen CA, Hawrylewicz EJ. Life in Extraterrestrial Environments. Chicago, IL, USA: Illinois Institute of Technology, 1962.

Hall R, Shayler D. The Rocket Men: Vostok and Voskhod, the First Manned Soviet Spaceflights. London, England: Springer, 2001.

Hanrahan JS, Bushnell D. Space Biology - The Human Factors in Space Flight. New York, NY, USA: Science Editions Inc, 1961.

Harding RM. Survival in Space - The Medical Problems of Manned Spaceflight. London - New York: Routledge, 1989.

Hardy JD. Physiological Problems in Space Exploration. Springfield IL, USA: Charles C. Thomas, 1964.

Hardy JD. Thermal Problems in Aerospace Medicine. London, England: Technical Publishing, 1968.

Harrison AA. Spacefaring: The Human Dimension. Berkeley, CA, USA: University of California Press, 2001.

Harrison AA, Clearwater YA. From Antarctica to Outer Space: Life in Isolation and Confinement. New York, NY, USA: Springer-Verlag, 1991.

Helvey W. Biomedical and Human Factors Requirements for a Manned Earth Orbiting Station. Farmindale, NY, USA: Republic Aviation Corporation, 1964.

Henry JP. Biomedical Aspects of Space Flight. New York, NY, USA: Holt, Rinehart and Winston Inc., 1966.

Hoyle F. Man in the Universe. New York, NY, USA: Columbia University Press, 1966.

Hoyle F, Wickramasinghe NC. Diseases from Space. New York, NY, USA: Harper & Row, 1991.

Huntoon CL. Humans in Spaceflight. Reston, VA, USA: American Institute of Aeronautics and Astronautics, 1997.

Huntoon CL, Grigor'ev AI. Fluid and Electrolyte Regulation in Spaceflight. San Diego, CA, USA: Univelt, 1998.

IAA Man in Space Symposium 1995. Man in Space for Science and Technology Development. England – USA: Pergamon Press, 1996.

Iazdovskii VI. Na Tropakh Vselennoi: Vklad Kosmicheskoi Biologii I Meditsiny v Osvoenie Kosmicheskogo Prostranstva. Moskva, Russia: Firma Slovo, 1996.

International Workshop on Cardiovascular Research in Space. International Workshop on Cardiovascular Research in Space: Dallas, Texas, September 1995. Indianapolis, IN, USA: American College of Sports Medicine, 1996.

Jenkins M. Human-Rating Requirements. Houston, TX, USA: Lyndon B. Johnson Space Center, 1998.

Johnson B, May GL. Humans and Machines in Space: The Vision, the Challenge, the Payoff. San Diego, CA, USA: Univelt, 1992.

Johnston RS, Dietlein LF. Biomedical Results from Skylab. NASA Special Publication # 377, Washington, DC, USA: U.S. Government Printing Office, 1977.

Johnston RS, Dietlein LF, Berry CA. Biomedical Results of Apollo. NASA Special Publication # 368, Washington, DC, USA: U.S. Government Printing Office, 1975.

Section III. Publications in Other Topics Related to Aerospace Medicine

Jones WJ, Simpson WC. NASA Contributions to Cardiovascular Monitoring. NASA Special Publication # 5041, Washington, DC, USA: U.S. Government Printing Office, 1966.

Kaldeich-Schurmann B. Sixth European Symposium on Life Sciences Research in Space: Proceedings, Trondheim, Norway June 1996. Noordwijk, Netherlands: European Space Agency Publications Division, 1996.

Kelly F. America's Astronauts and Their Indestructible Spirit. Blue Ridge, PA, USA: 1986.

Kinney WA. Medical Science and Space Travel. New York, NY, USA: F. Watts, 1959.

Klein KE, Contant JM. Living and Working in Space: A Selection of Papers Presented at the 9th IAA Man in Space Symposium, Cologne, Germany, June 1991. England – USA: Pergamon Press, 1992.

Koltun EA, Giurdzhian AA. Mediko-Biologicheskie I Sotsial'no-Psikhologicheskie Problemy Kosmicheskikh Poletov. Moskva, USSR: Izd-vo Nauka, 1978.

Konecci EB. Manned Space Cabin Systems. Santa Monica, CA, USA: Douglas Aircraft Company, 1959.

Konstantinova IV, Fuchs BB. The Immune System in Space and Other Extreme Conditions. England – USA: Harwood Academic Publishers, 1991.

Kranz G. Failure is Not an Option: Mission Control from Mercury to Apollo 13 and Beyond. New York, NY, USA: Simon & Schuster, 2000.

Krylova NV, Ratner GS. Materialy XXI Gagarinskikh Nauchnykh Chtenii po Aviatsii I Kosmonavtike: Sektsiia Problemy Aviakosmicheskoi Meditsiny i Psikhologii. Moskva, USSR: In-t Psikhologii, 1991.

Lamb LE. Aeromedical Evaluation for Space Pilots. San Antonio, TX, USA: USAF School of Aerospace Medicine, Brooks AFB, 1963.

Landeau J. Espace et Mer. Paris, France: European Space Agency, 1990.

Lane HW, Schoeller DA. Nutrition in Spaceflight and Weightlessness Models. Boca Raton, FL, USA: CRC Press, 1999.

Langham WH. Radiobiological Factors in Manned Space Flight. Washington, DC, USA: National Academy of Sciences, 1967.

Langley Research Center. Research in Aeronautics and Space. Washington, DC, USA: U.S. Government Printing Office, 1971.

Lansberg MP. A Primer of Space Medicine. New York, NY, USA: Elsevier, 1960.

Larson W, Pranke LK. Human Spaceflight: Mission Analysis and Design. New York, NY, USA: McGraw-Hill, 2000.

Lavnikov AA. Osnovy Aviatsionnoi I Kosmocheskoi Meditsiny. Moskva: USSR: Voennoe Izd-vo Ministerstva Oborony SSSF, 1975.

Lent HB. Man Alive in Outer Space. New York, NY, USA: The MacMillan Co., 1961.

Lindsey JF, Townsend JC. Biomedical Research and Computer Application in Manned Space Flight. NASA Special Publication # 5078, Washington, DC, USA: U.S. Government Printing Office, 1971.

Link MM. Space Medicine in Project Mercury. NASA Special Publication # 4003, Washington, DC, USA: U.S. Government Printing Office, 1965.

Looney JJ. Bibliography of Space Books and Articles from Non-Aerospace Journals, 1957-1977. Washington, DC, USA: U.S. Government Printing Office, 1979.

Lorr DB, Garshnek V, Cadoux C. Working in Orbit and Beyond: The Challenges for Space Medicine. San Diego, CA, USA: Univelt Inc., 1989.

Malone TB, Bender HE, Kahn MH. An Analysis of Astronaut Performance Capability in the Lunar Environment. Alexandria, VA, USA: Matrix, 1969.

Marbarger JP. Space Medicine: The Human Factors in Flights Beyond the Earth. Urbana IL, USA: University of Illinois Press, 1951.

McCally M. Hypodynamics and Hypogravics. New York - London: Academic Press Inc., 1968.

McCally M, Murray RH. Hypogravic and Hypodynamic Environments. NASA Special Publication # 269, Washington, DC, USA: U.S. Government Printing Office, 1969.

McNamara B. Into the Final Frontier: The Human Exploration of Space. England – USA: Harcourt College, 2001.

Mikhailova NN, Koltun EA. Mediko-Biologischeskie I Sotsail'no Psikhologischeskie Problemy Osvoeniia Kosmosa I Regionov Zemli s Ekstremal'nymi Usloviiami Sushchestvovaniaa. Moskva, USSR: Nauka, 1987.

Montemerlo MD, Cron AC. Space Human Factors: Workshop Proceedings. McLean, VA, USA: General Research Corporation, 1982.

Moore D, Bie P. Biological and Medical Research in Space: An Overview of Life Sciences Research in Microgravity. Germany – USA: Springer-Verlag, 1996.

Moskalenko UE, Kas'ian II. Vnutricherepnoe Krovoobrashchenie v Usloviiakh Peregruzok I Nevesomosti. Moskva, USSR: Meditsina, 1971.

Müller B. Die Gesamte Luftfahrt und Raumflugmedizin. Düsseldorf, Germany: Ministerium für Wirtschaft, 1967.

Müller B. Raumfahrtmedizin: Kompendium der Raumfahrtmedizin. Druck, Germany: Droste Verlag, 1963.

Napolitano LG. Space – Mankind's Fourth Environment. England – USA: Pergamon Press, 1982.

National Academy of Sciences. Physiology in the Space Environment. Washington, DC, USA: U.S. Government Printing Office, 1967.

National Aeronautics and Space Administration. Aerospace Medicine and Biology: A Continuing Bibliography with Indexes. NASA Special Publication # 7011.

National Aeronautics and Space Administration. First Conference on the Role of the Vestibular Organs in the Exploration of Space. NASA Special Publication # 77, Washington, DC, USA: U.S. Government Printing Office, 1965.

National Aeronautics and Space Administration. Second Symposium on the Role of the Vestibular Organs in Space Exploration. NASA Special Publication # 115, Washington, DC, USA: U.S. Government Printing Office, 1966.

National Aeronautics and Space Administration. Third Symposium on the Role of the Vestibular Organs in Space Exploration. NASA Special Publication # 152, Washington, DC, USA: U.S. Government Printing Office, 1967.

National Aeronautics and Space Administration. Fourth Symposium on the Role of the Vestibular Organs in Space Exploration. NASA Special Publication # 187, Washington, DC, USA: U.S. Government Printing Office, 1968.

National Aeronautics and Space Administration. Fifth Symposium on the Role of the Vestibular Organs in Space Exploration. NASA Special Publication # 314, Washington, DC, USA: U.S. Government Printing Office, 1970.

National Aeronautics and Space Administration. Medical and Biological Applications of Space Telemetry. NASA Special Publication # 5023, Washington, DC, USA: U.S. Government Printing Office, 1965.

National Aeronautics and Space Administration. Records of Achievement: NASA Special Publications. Washington, DC, USA: U.S. Government Printing Office, 1983.

National Aeronautics and Space Administration. Biomedicine - A Compilation. NASA Special Publication # 5958. Washington, DC, USA: U.S. Government Printing Office, 1973.

National Aeronautics and Space Administration, Life Sciences Strategic Planning Study Committee. Exploring The Living Universe - A Strategy For Space Life Sciences. Washington, DC, USA: U.S. Government Printing Office, 1988.

National Aeronautics and Space Administration, Scientific and Technical Information Branch. Life Sciences Accomplishments. NASA Technical Memorandum # 88177, Washington, DC, USA: U.S. Government Printing Office, 1985.

National Aeronautics and Space Administration, Terrestrial Applications Program, Technology Utilization Division. Bioengineering and Rehabilitation - Windows of Opportunity Past, Present and Future. NASA Special Publication # EP-216, Washington, DC, USA: U.S. Government Printing Office, 1985.

National Council on Radiation Protection and Measurements. Accepatability of Risk from Radiation: Application to Human Space Flight. Bethesda, MD, USA: National Council on Radiation Protection and Measurements, 1997.

National Council on Radiation Protection and Measurements. Radiation Protection Guidance for Activities in Low-Earth Orbit. Bethesda, MD, USA: National Council on Radiation Protection and Measurements, 2000.

National Research Council, Committee on Space Biology and Medicine, Space Studies Board. A Strategy for Research in Space Biology and Medicine into the Next Century. Washington, DC, USA: National Academy Press, 1998.

National Research Council, Committee on Space Biology and Medicine, Space Studies Board. Review of NASA's Biomedical Research Program. Washington, DC, USA: National Academy Press, 2000.

Section III. Publications in Other Topics Related to Aerospace Medicine

National Research Council, Space Studies Board. The Human Exploration of Space. Washington, DC, USA: National Academy Press, 1997.

National Research Council, Space Studies Board. Report of the Workshop on Biology-Based Technology to Enhance Human Well-Being and Function in Extended Space Exploration. Washington, DC, USA: National Academy Press, 1998.

National Research Council, Task Group on the Biological Effects of Space Radiation, Space Studies Board. Radiation Hazards to Crews of Interplanetary Missions: Biological Issues and Research Strategies. Washington, DC, USA: National Academy Press, 1996.

Nemere I. Halottak Keringenek a Kozmoszban: Kozmikus Hazugságok: A Szovjet Urkutatás Titkai. Budapest, Hungary, ALTER-NATÍV, 1998.

Nicogossian AE. The Apollo-Soyuz Test Project Medical Report. NASA Special Publication # 411, Washington, DC, USA: U.S. Government Printing Office, 1977.

Nicogossian AE. Space Biology and Medicine. Washington, DC, USA: American Institute of Aeronautics and Astronautics; Moscow, Russia: Nauka, 1993.

Nicogossian AE, Huntoon CL. Space Physiology and Medicine. Philadelphia, PA, USA: Lea & Febiger, 1994.

Nicogossian AE, Hunton CL, Pool SL. Space Physiology and Medicine. 2nd Edition, Philadelphia - London - England: Lea & Febiger, 1989.

Nicogossian AE, Parker Jr JF. Space Physiology and Medicine. Washington, DC, USA: U.S. Government Printing Office, NASA Special Publication # 447, 1983.

Nieto Boque M. Vida Humana y Espacio: Medicina Cosmonáutica. Barcelona, Spain: Editorial Jims, 1965.

Oberth H. Menschen im Weltraum. Dusseldorf, Econ. English translation: Man Into Space. New York, NY, USA: Harper, 1954.

Oman CM. Space Motion Sickness and Vestibular Experiments in Spacelab. Warrendale, PA, USA: Society of Automotive Engineers, 1982.

Parker JF, West VR. Biostronautics Data Book. Washington, DC, USA: U. S. Government Printing Office, 1973.

Peters RA. Dynamics of the Vestibular System and their Relation to Motion Perception, Spatial Disorientation and Illusions. NASA-CR-1309, Washington, DC, USA: U. S. Government Printing Office, 1969.

Pitts JAS. The Human Factor: Biomedicine in the Manned Space Program to 1980. NASA Scientific and Technical Information Branch, Washington, DC, USA: U.S. Government Printing Office, 1985.

Popovich P, Gubinskii AI. Ergonomicheskoe Obespechenie Deiatel'nosti Kosmonatov. Moskva, Russia: Mashinostroenie, 1985.

Reimer T. Die Entwicklung der Flugmedizin in Deutschland. Köln, Germany: F. Hansen, 1979.

Rivolier J. L'Homme dans l'Espace: une Approche Psycho-Écologique des Vols Habités. Paris, France: Presses Universitaires de France, 1997.

Roos C. Bibliography of Space Medicine. Washington, DC, USA: National Library of Medicine, 1958.

Roth EM. Compendium of Human Responses to the Aerospace Environment. NASA Contractor Report No. CR-1205, Washington, DC, USA: U. S. Government Printing Office, 1968.

Sandler H, Winter DL. Physiological Responses of Women to Simulated Weightlessness. NASA Special Publication # 430. Washington, DC, USA: U.S. Government Printing Office, 1978.

Santy PA. Choosing the Right Stuff: The Psychological Selection of Astronauts and Cosmonauts. Westport, CT, USA: Praeger, 1994.

Scano A, Strollo F. Life Sciences Experiments in Space Bring Benefits on Earth. Noordwijk, Netherlands: ESA Publications Division, 1997.

Schaefer KF. Bioastronautics. New York, NY, USA: The Macmillan Co., 1964.

Schaefer KE. Man's Dependence on the Earthly Astosphere. New York, NY, USA: Macmillan, 1962.

Sekiguchi C. Uchu Igaku, Seirigaku. Tokyo, Japan: Shakai Hoken Shuppansha, 1998.

Sharpe MR. Living in Space - the Astronaut and his Environment. Garden City, USA: Doubleday, 1969.

Shayler D. Disasters and Accidents in Manned Spaceflight. London, England: Springer, 2000.

Simons DG. Man High. Garden City, NJ, USA: 1960.

Sisakian NM, Gazenko OG. Pervaia Kosmicheskaia Laboratoriia: Rezultaty Mediko-Biologicheskikh Issledovanii Poleta Korablia "Voskhod." Moskva, USSR: Izdateastvo Nauka, 1966.

Slager UT. Space Medicine. London, England: Prentice Hall, 1962.

Smirnov KV. Kosmicheskaia Gastroenterologiia: Trofologicheskie Ocherki. Moskva, USSR: Nauka, 1981.

Sokov VS. Space Flight and Aeromedicine: General Survey with Research Subject Directory and Bibliography. 1st Edition, Washington, DC, USA: ABBE Publishers Association of Washington, DC, 1983.

Souza KA, Etheridge G. Life Into Space: Space Life Sciences Experiments, Ames Research Center, Kennedy Space Center, 1991-1998. Washington DC, USA: U.S. Government Printing Office, 2000.

Stahle J. Vestibular Function on Earth and in Space. Oxford - London: Pergamon Press, 1970.

Stuster J. Bold Endeavors: Lessons from Polar and Space Exploration. Annapolis, MD, USA: Naval Institute Press, 1996.

Swenberg CE, Horneck G. Biological Effects and Physics of Solar and Galactic Cosmic Radiation. New York, NY, USA: Plenum Press, 1993.

Tabusse L, Pannier R. Physiopathologie et pathologie Aéronautiques et Cosmonautiques. Paris, France: Doin, Deren et Cie, 1969.

Taylor ER. Physical and Physiological Data for Bioastronautics. Randolph AFB, TX, USA: USAF School of Aviation Medicine, 1958.

Thomas S. Men of Space. New York, NY, USA: Hillman Books, 1961.

Thompson AB. Physiological and Psychological Considerations for Manned Space Flight. Dallas, TX, USA: Chance Vought Aircraft Inc., 1959.

U.S. Office of Manned Space Flight. A Review of Medical Results of Gemini 7 and Related Flights. Washington, DC, USA: U.S. Government Printing Office, 1966.

Uskov FN, Simonov PV. Distantsionnoe Nabliudenie I Ekspertnaia Otsenka: Obshchenie I Kommunikatsiia v Zadachakh Meditsinskogo Kontrolia. Moskva, USSR: Izd-vo Nauka, 1982.

Vasil'eva VV. Gazenko OG. Mediko-Biologicheskie I Sotsial'no-Psikhologicheskie Problemy Osvoeniia Kosmosa I Regionov Zemli s Ekstremal'nymi Usloviiami Sushchestvovaniia. Moskva, Russia: Rossilskaia Akademiia Nauk, 1992.

Vinograd SP. Medical Aspects of an Orbiting Research Laboratory. NASA Special Publication # 86, Washington, DC, USA: U.S. Government Printing Office, 1964.

Volynkin IM. The First Manned Space Flights. Dayton, OH, USA: Air Force Systems Command, 1962.

Wachhorst W. The Dream of Spaceflight: Essays on the Near Edge of Infinity. New York, NY, USA: Basic Books, 2000.

Waligora. The Physiological Basis for Spacecraft Environmental Limits. NASA Special Publication # 1045, Washington, DC, USA: U.S. Government Printing Office, 1979.

Wang T. Chung I Yu Hang Ping Hsueh. Hsi-an, China: Shen-hsi K'o Hsueh Chi Shu Ch'u Pan She, 1996.

Watanabe S, Yajima K. At the Threshold of the 21st Century: A Selection of Papers Presented at the 10th IAA Man in Space Symposium, Tokyo, Japan, April 1993. England – New York: Pergamon Press, 1994.

Webb P. Bioatronautics Data Book. NASA Special Publication # 3006, Washington, DC, USA: U.S. Government Printing Office, 1964.

Weltman G. NASA Contributions to Bioinstrumentation Systems. Washington, DC, USA: U.S. Government Printing Office, NASA Special Publication # 5054, 1968.

Whitmore M, McQuilkin ML. Habitability and Performance Issues for Long Duration Space Flights. Washington, DC, USA: National Aeronautics and Space Administration, 1997.

Willmore AP, Willmore SR. Aerospace Research Index: A Guide to World Research in Aeronautics, Meteorology, Astronomy, and Space Science. England – USA: Gale Research Company, 1981.

Wunder CG. Life into Space - An Introduction to Space Biology. Philadelphia, PA, USA: F. A. Davies, 1966.

Yegorov AD. Results of Medical Research during the 175-day Flight of the Third Prime Crew on the Salyut-6 Soyuz Orbital Complex. Washington, DC, USA: U.S. Government Printing Office, NASA Technical Memorandum # 76450, 1980.

Yegorov AD. Results of Medical Studies during Long-Term Manned Flights on the Orbital Salyut-6 and Soyuz Complex. Washington, DC, USA: U.S. Government Printing Office, NASA Technical Memorandum # 76014, 1979.

Section III. Publications in Other Topics Related to Aerospace Medicine

Diving Physiology and Medicine

Adolfson J, Berhage T. Perception and Performance Under Water. New York, NJ, USA: Wiley, 1974.

Aerospace Technology Division. Soviet Naval Medicine and Underwater Physiology. Washington DC, USA: Library of Congress, 1968.

Albano G. Principles and Observations on the Physiology of the Scuba Diver. Washington, DC, USA: Superintendent of Documents, U.S. Government Printing Office, 1970.

Bachrach AJ, Egstrom GH. Stress and Performance in Diving. San Pedro, CA, USA: Best Publishing Co., 1987.

Beljan JR, Hellwell AB. Medical Applications of Space Related Research: Calcium and Bone. Davis, CA, USA: University of California, 1973.

Bennett PB, Elliott DH. The Physiology and Medicine of Diving. England – USA: Saunders, 1993.

Bennett PB, Elliott DH. The Physiology and Medicine of Diving. London, England: Bailliere Tindall, 1982.

Bennett PB, Elliott DH. The Physiology and Medicine of Diving and Compressed Air Work. Baltimore, MD, USA: Williams and Wilkins Co., 1969.

Bernard T. Medicine de la Plongee - Medicine Hyperbare Professionnelle et Sportive. Paris - New York: Masson, 1982.

Bookspan JN. Diving Physiology in Plain English. Kensington, MD, USA: Undersea and Hyperbaric Society, 1995.

Bove AA, Davis JC. Diving Medicine. Philadelphia, PA, USA: W.B. Saunders Co., 1990.

Buhlmann AA. Decompression-Decompression Sickness. Berlin - Hiedelberg - New York - Tokyo: Springer-Verlag, 1984.

Buhlmann AA. Tauchmedizin: Barotauma, Gasembolie, Dekompression, Dekompressionskrankheit. Germany – USA: Springer-Verlag, 1993.

Burnazzian AI, Gazenko OG. Spravochnik po Kosmicheskoi Biologii I Meditsine. Moskva, USSR: Meditsina, 1983.

Busch WS. Safety and Medical Considerations in Diving. Washington, DC, USA: Marine Technology Society, 1989.

Chauchard P. La Vie en Vol et en Plongee; de L'Astronef au Bathyscaphe. Paris, France: A. Michel, 1958.

Chernigovskii VN, Vasilev PV. Patofiziologicheskie osnovy Aviatsionnoi I Kosmicheskoi. Moskva, USSR: Nauka, 1971.

Committee on Hyperbaric Oxygenation, National Academy of Sciences/National Research Council. Fundamentals of Hyperbaric Medicine. Washington, DC, USA: U.S. Government Printing Office, 1966.

Crockett PW. Underwater Medicine and Physiology: A Bibliography with Abstracts. Springfield, VA, USA: National Technical Information Service, 1976.

Davis JC. Medical Examination of Sport Scuba Divers. San Pedro, CA, USA: Best Publishing Co., 1986.

Davis JC, Bove AA. Diving Medicine. San Pedro, CA, USA: Best Publishing Co., 1989.

Davis JC, Hunt TK. Hyperbaric Oxygen Therapy. Bethesda, MD, USA: Undersea Medical Society, 1977.

Davis JC, Hunt TK. Problem Wounds. The role of Oxygen. San Pedro, CA, USA: Best Publishing Co., 1988.

Dueker CW. Scuba Diving in Safety and Health. San Pedro, CA, USA: Best Publishing Co., 1984.

Dueker CW. Medical Aspects of Sport Diving. South Brunswick, NJ, USA: A. S. Barnes, 1970.

Eastmen PF. Advanced First Aid Afloat. San Pedro, CA, USA: Best Publishing Co., 1979.

Edmonds C. Otological Aspects of Diving. Glebe, Australia: Australasian Medical Publications Co., 1973.

Edmonds C, Lowry C. Diving and Subaquatic Medicine. England – USA: Butterworth-Heinemann, 1992.

Edmonds C, Lowry C, Pennefather J. Diving and Subaquatic Medicine. California, USA: Best Publishing Co., 1981.

Edmonds C, McKenzie B. Diving Medicine for Scuba Divers. Carnegie, Victoria, Australia: J. L. Publications, 1992.

Elsner BG, Gooden B. Diving and Asphyxia: A Comparative Study of Animals and Man. Cambridge, NJ, USA: Cambridge University Press, 1983.

Fife W. Women in Diving: Proceedings of the Thirty-Fifth Undersea and Hyperbaric Medical Society Workshop, Bethesda, Maryland, 1986. Bethesda, MD, USA: Undersea and Hyperbaric Medical Society, 1987.

Fisher AA. Atlas of Aquatic Dermatology. New York, NJ, USA: Grune & Stratton, 1978.

Francis TJR, Smith DJ. Describing Decompression Illness: Proceedings of the Forty-Second Workshop of the Undersea and Hyperbaric Medical Society, Hampshire, UK, 1990. Bethesda, MD, USA: Undersea and Hyperbaric Medical Society, 1991.

Fructus, Sciarli R. La Plongee: Sante, Securite. Paris, France: Editions Maritimes et D'Outre Mer, 1980.

Fulton JF. Decompression Sickness, Caisson Sickness, Diver's and Flier's Bends and Related Syndromes. Philadelphia, PA, USA: W. B. Saunders Co., 1957.

Gallar F. Medicina Subacuática e Hiperbárica. Madrid, Spain: Instituto Social de la Marina, 1987.

Gatland KW. Manned Spacecraft. New York, NY, USA: Macmillan, 1976.

Gilliam B, Von Maier R. Deep Diving: An Advanced Guide to Physiology, Procedures and Systems. San Diego, CA, USA: Watersport Publishing, 1995.

Goethe WHG, Watson EN, Jones DT. Handbook of Nautical Medicine. New York, NY, USA: Springer-Verlag, 1984.

Guyton AC. Physiology of Deep Sea Diving and Other High-Pressure Operations. In: Textbook of Medical Physiology, Philadelphia - London - Toronto: W.B. Saunders Company, 1981;552-558.

Hempleman HV, Lockwood AP. The Physiology of Diving in Man and other Animals. London, England: E. Arnold, 1978.

Hendrick W, Thomson B. Oxygen and the Scuba Diver. San Pedro, CA, USA: Best Publishing Co., 1988.

Hill L. Caisson Disease. New York, NJ, USA: Longmans, Green & Co., Inc., 1912.

Hills BA. Decompression Sickness: The Biophysical Basis of Prevention and Treatment. London - New York: Wiley, 1977.

Hoff EC, Greenbaum LJ. A Bibliographical Sourcebook of Compressed Air, Diving, and Submarine Medicine. Washington, DC, USA: U.S. Government Printing Office, 1948.

Hong SK. International Symposium on Man in the Sea. Bethesda, MD, USA: Undersea Medical Society, 1975.

Kinney JAS. Human Underwater Vision: Physiology and Physics. Bethesda, MD, USA: Undersea Medical Society, 1985.

Kisliakov UA, Breslav KS. Dykhanie, Dinamika Gazov I Rabotosposobnost'pri Giperbarii. Leningrad, USSR: Nauka, 1988.

Kolchinskaia AZ. Podvodnye Mediko-Fiziologicheskie Issledovaniia. Kiev, USSSR: Akademiia Nauk URSR - Institut Fiziologii, 1975.

Kreps EM, Zal'tsman GL. Organizm v Usloviiakh Dlitel'noi Giperbarii. Kiev, USSSR: Akademiia Nauk URSR - Institut Evoliutsionnoi Fiziologii i Biokhimii, 1977.

Lambertsen CJ. Underwater Physiology. New York, NY, USA: Academic Press, 1971.

Lanphier EH, Rahn H. Man, Water, Pressure: Publications in Underwater Physiology. Buffalo, NY, USA: State University of New York, 1966.

Lederer RJ. Medicine et Plongee. Paris, France: Editions Maritimes et d'outre-mer, 1973.

Lewbell GS. The Decompression Workbook. San Pedro, CA, USA: Best Publishing Co., 1984.

Lin YC, Niu AKC. Hyperbaric Physiology and Medicine. San Pedro, CA, USA: Best Publishing Co., 1988.

Lin YC, Shida KK. Man in The Sea. San Pedro, CA, USA: Best Publishing Co.,1990.

Mandojana RM. Aquatic Dermatology. Philadelphia, PA, USA: Lippincott, 1987.

Marroni A. Il Medico Sott'acqua. Firenze, Italy: Olimpia, 1974.

Martin L. Scuba Diving Explained: Questions and Answers on Physiology and Medical Aspects of Scuba Diving. Flagstaff, AZ, USA: Best Publishing Company, 1997.

Matthys H. Medizinische Tauchfibel. Berlin - New York: Springer Verlag, 1978.

Miles S. Underwater Medicine. London, England: Staples P., 1969.

Miles S, Mackay DE. Underwater Medicine. Philadelphia, PA, USA: Lippincott, 1976.

Miller JW. Visual Problems of Space Travel. Washington, DC, USA: National Academy of Sciences, 1962.

Molfino F, Zannini D. L'Uomo e il Mondo Sommerso; Medicina Subacquea. Torino, Italy: Minerva Medica, 1964.

Nashimoto I. Kaitei ni Sumu. Japan: 1971.

Nashimoto I, Lanphier EH. What is Bends?: Proceedings of the Forty-Third Undersea and Hyperbaric Medical Society Workshop, Shimizu, Japan, November 1990. Bethesda, MD, USA: Undersea and Hyperbaric Medical Society, 1991.

Section III. Publications in Other Topics Related to Aerospace Medicine

National Research Council – Committee on Undersea Warfare. Status of Research in Underwater Physiology. Washington, DC, USA: National Academy of Sciences, 1956.

Nelson J, Brebner J. The Offshore Health Handbook - A practical guide to coping with injury and illness. San Pedro, CA, USA: Best Publishing Co., 1985.

Phillips JL. The Bends: Compressed Air in the History of Science, Diving, and Engineering. New Haven, CT, USA: Yale University Press, 1998.

Radloff R, Helmreich R. Groups Under Stress - Psychological Research in SEALAB II. New York, NJ, USA: Appleton-Century-Crofts, 1968.

Rahn H, Yokoyama T. Physiology of Breath-Hold Diving and the Ama of Japan. Washington, DC, USA: National Academy of Sciences-National Research Council, 1965.

Reilly RE. Human Performance in the Undersea Environment. Detroit, MI, USA: Management Information Services, 1969.

Roydhouse N. Scuba Diving and the Ear, Nose, and Throat. Auckland, New Zealand, 1973.

Roydhouse N. Underwater Ear & Nose Care. San Pedro, CA, USA: Best Publishing Co., 1981.

Roydhouse N. Underwater Ear & Nose Care. Flagstaff, AZ, USA: Best Publishing Co., 1993.

Schaefer KE. Preventive Aspects of Submarine Medicine. Bethesda, MD, USA: Undersea Medical Society, 1979.

Sheffield PJ. Flying After Diving: Proceedings of the Thirty-Ninth Undersea and Hyperbaric Medical Society, Bethesda, Maryland, February 1989. Bethesda, MD, USA: Undersea and Hyperbaric Medical Society, 1989.

Sheffield PJ, Moon RE. Treatment of Decompression Illness: Proceedings of the Forty-Fifth Undersea and Hyperbaric Medical Society Workshop, Palm Beach, Florida, June 1995. Kensington, MD, USA: Undersea and Hyperbaric Medical Society, 1996.

Shilling CW, Carlston CB, Mathias RA. Physician's Guide to Diving Medicine. New York; Plenum Press, 1984.

Shilling CW, Werts MF. An Annotated Bibliography on Diving and Submarine Medicine. New York, NJ, USA: Gordon & Breach. 1971.

Shilling CW, Werts MF. The Underwater Handbook: A Guide to Physiology and Performance for the Engineer. London, England: Wiley, 1976.

Shilling CW, Werst MF. Underwater Medicine and Related Sciences: A Guide to the Literature: An Annotated Bibliography, Key Word Index, and Microthesaurus. New York, NY, USA: IFI/Plenum, 1973.

Shiraki K, Yousef MK. Man in Stressful Environments: Diving, Hyper- and Hypobaric Physiology. Springfield, IL, USA: Charles C. Thomas, 1987.

Smith NE, Hotta H. Proceedings of the 14th Meeting of the United States-Japan Cooperative Program in Natural Resources: Panel on Diving Physiology. Panama City, Florida, September 1997. Washington, DC, USA: U.S. Government Printing Office, 1998.

Soviet Naval Medicine and Underwater Physiology. Washington, DC, USA: U.S. Library of Congress - Aerospace Technology Division, 1968.

Strauss RH. Diving Medicine. New York, NJ, USA: Grune & Stratton, 1976.

Thomas R, McKenzie B. The Diver's Medical Companion. San Pedro, CA, USA: Best Publishing Co., 1981.

Thomas RS. Choice of an Atmosphere for an Extended Space Mission. Sunnyvale, CA, USA: Lockhead Missiles & Space Company, 1963.

Trimble VH. The Uncertain Miracle - Hyperbaric Oxygenation. Garden City, USA: Doubleday, 1974.

Undersea and Hyperbaric Medical Society. Hyperbaric Chambers, United States and Canada: A Directory of Hyperbaric Treatment Chambers, Hyperbaric Oxygen Therapy, Decompression Sickness Therapy. Kensington, MD, USA: Undersea and Hyperbaric Medical Society, 1997.

Undersea Medical Society. Key Documents of the Biomedical Aspects of Deep-Sea Diving; Selected from the World's Literature (1608-1982). Bethesda, MD, USA: Undersea Medical Society, 1983.

Vann RD. The Physiological Basis of Decompression: Proceedings of the Thirty-Eighth Undersea and Hyperbaric Medical Society Workshop, Duke University Medical Center, 1987. Bethesda, MD, USA: Undersea and Hyperbaric Medical Society, 1987.

Verjano Díaz F. El Hombre Subacuático: Manual de Fisiología y Riesgos del Buceo. Madrid, Spain: Díaz de Santos, 2000.

Vorosmarti J, Linaweaver PG. Fitness to Dive: Proceedings of the Thirty-Fourth Undersea and Hyperbaric Medical Workshop, Bethesda, Maryland, May 1986. Bethesda, MD, USA: Undersea and Hyperbaric Medical Society, 1987.

White WJ. A Survey of Bioastronautics 1961-1962. Buffalo, NY, USA: Cornell Aeronautical Laboratory, 1962.

Wienke BR. Basic Decompression Theory and Application. Flagstaff, AZ, USA: Best Publishing Company, 1991.

Wienke BR. Diving Above Sea Level. Flagstaff, AZ, USA: Best Publishing Company, 1993.

Wienke BR. High Altitude Diving. Montclair, CA, USA: National Association of Underwater Instructors, 1992.

Wu WL. Human Factors Standards for the Apollo Program. Albuquerque, NM, USA: Lovelace Foundation, 1965.

Aerospace Human Factors and Psychology

Abeyratne RI. Aviation Trends in the New Millennium. England – USA: Ashgate, 2001.

Advisory Group for Aeronautical Research & Development. Methods and Criteria for the Selection of Flying Personnel. Paris, France: AGARD, 1954.

Advisory Group for Aerospace Research & Development. A Designer's Guide to Human Performance Modelling. Neuilly-sur-Seine, France: AGARD, 1998.

Amalberti R. Facteurs Humains. Rungis, France: Institut Aéronautique Jean Mermoz, 1996.

Anderson N, Peiper H. Eliminating Pilot Error: The Final Step in Flight Training. East Cannan, CT, USA: ATN Publishing, 1999.

Baldwin R. Developing the Future Aviation System. England – USA: Ashgate, 1998.

Beaty D. The Naked Pilot: The Human Factor in Aircraft Accidents. Shrewsbury, England: Airlife, 1995.

Billings CE. Aviation Automation: The Search for a Human-Centered Approach. Mahwah, NJ, USA: Lawrence Erlbaum Associates Publishers, 1997.

Billings CE, Eggspuehler JJ, Gerke R. Studies of Pilot Performance in the Flight Environment. Columbus, OH, USA: Ohio State University Press, 1966.

Buck RN. The Pilot's Burden: Flight Safety and the Roots of Pilot Error. Ames, IA, USA: Iowa State University, 2000.

Campbell RD, Bagshaw M. Human Performance and Limitations in Aviation. England – USA: BSP Professional Books, 1991.

Campbell RD, Bagshaw M. Human Performance and Limitations in Aviation. England – USA: Blackwell Science, 1999.

Cheston TS, Winter DL. Human Factors of Outer Space Production. USA: American Association for the Advancement of Science, 1980.

Cohen SI, Silverman AJ. Measurement of Pilot Mental Effort. Paris, France: North Atlantic Treaty Organization (NATO), 1957.

Cohn RL. They Called It Pilot Error: True Stories Behind General Aviation Accidents. New York, NY, USA: TAB Books, 1994.

Collins RL. Air Crashes: What Went Wrong, Why, and What Can Be Done About It. Charlottesville, VA, USA: Thomasson-Grant, 1992.

Craig PA. The Killing Zone: How and Why Pilots Die. New York, NY, USA: McGraw-Hill, 2001.

Dahlberg A. Air Rage: The Underestimated Safety Risk. England – USA: Ashgate, 2001.

Davis DR. Pilot Error: Some Laboratory Experiments. London, England: His Majesty's Stationery Office, 1948.

Davis M. Through the Stratosphere - The Human Factor in Aviation. New York, NY, USA: The Macmillan Co., 1946.

Deitz SR, Thoms WE. Pilots, Personality, and Performance: Human Behavoir and Stress in the Skies. New York, NY, USA: Quorum Books, 1991.

Dekker S, Hollnagel E. Coping with Computers in the Cockpit. Brookfield, VT, USA: Ashgate, 1999.

Dissfeldt H. Bewährungskontrolle Eines Psychologischen Auswahlverfahrens für den Flugverkehrskontrolldienst Anhand von Kriterien der Berufsausbildung. Köln, Germany: Deutsche Forschungsanstalt für Luft-und Raumfahrt, 1991.

Doll RE, Berkshire JR. Psychological Research in the U.S. Naval School of Aviation Medicine, 1950-1960. Pensacola, FL, USA: U.S. Naval School of Aviation Medicine.

Edwards DC. Pilot: Mental and Physical Performance. Ames, IA, USA: Iowa State University Press, 1990.

Edwards M, Edwards E. The Aircraft Cabin - Managing the Human Factors. Brookfield, VT, USA: Gower Publishing Company, 1990.

Elizalde O. Factores humanos I: Aspectos Psicosociales del Fallo Humano en los Accidentes. Madrid, Spain, IBERIA, 1985.

Section III. Publications in Other Topics Related to Aerospace Medicine

Emeyriat B. Facteurs humains en Sécurité Aérienne. Mont-Royal, Québec: Modulo, 1997.

Endsley MR, Garland DJ. Situation Awareness: Analysis and Measurement. Mahwah, NJ, USA: Lawrence Erlbaum Associates Publishers, 2000.

Farmer E. Handbook of Simulator-Based Training. England – USA: Ashgate, 1999.

Farmer E. Human Resource Management in Aviation. Brookfield, VT, USA: Avebury Technical, 1991.

Farmer E. Stress and Error in Aviation. Brookfield, VT, USA: Avebury Technical, 1991.

Flanagan JC. The Aviation Psychology Program in the Army Air Forces. Washington, DC, USA: U.S. Government Printing Office, 1948.

Flying Magazine. Pilot Error: Anatomies of Aircraft Accidents. New York, NY, USA: Van Nostrand Reinhold, 1977.

Freeman F, Goshen CE, King BG. The Role of Human Factors in Accident Prevention. Washington, DC, USA: Department of Health, Education and Welfare, 1960.

Gallagher RD, De Remer D. Human Factors and Crew Resource Management for Flight Instructors: The New Student Involvement. Grand Fords, ND, USA: Eastern Dakota Publishers, 1993.

Garland DJ, Wise JA. Handbook of Aviaton Human Factors. Mahwah, NJ, USA: Lawrence Erlbaum Associates Publishers, 1999.

Garland DJ, Wise JA. Human Factors and Advanced Aviation Technologies. Daytona Beach, FL, USA: Embry Riddle Aeronautical University Press, 1993.

Goeters KM. Aviation Psychology: A Science and a Profession. England – USA: Ashgate, 1998.

Green RG. Human Factors for Pilots. England – USA: Ashgate, 1996.

Green RG, Muir H, Gradwell D, Green RL, James M. Human Factors for Pilots. Brookfield, VT, USA: Avebury Technical, 1991

Green RJ, Self HC. 50 Years of Human Engineering: History and Cumulative Bibliography of the Fitts Human Engineering Division. Springfield, VA, USA: National Technical Information Service, 1995.

Harris D. Engineering Psychology and Cognitive Ergonomics, 4 volumes. England – USA: Ashgate, 1997-1999.

Hawkins FH. Human Factors in Flight. England - USA: Gower Technical Press, 1987.

Hawkins FH, Orlady HW. Human Factors in Flight. Aldershot, England: Ashgate, 1993.

Helmreich RL, Merritt AC. Culture at Work in Aviation and Medicine: National, Organizational, and Professional Influences. England – USA: Ashgate, 1998.

Herrero Aldama P. Problemas Psiquiátricos in Aeronáutica. Madrid, Spain: Ejercito del Aire, 1982.

Hopkin VD. Human Factors in Air Traffic Control. England – USA: Taylor & Francis, 1995.

Hunt GJF. Designing Instruction for Human Factors Training in Aviation. England – USA: Avebury Aviation, 1997.

Hunter DR, Burke EF. Handbook of Pilot Selection. England – USA: Avebury Aviation, 1995.

Hurst K, Hurst L. Pilot Error - The Human Factors. New York, NY, USA: Jason Aronson, 1982.

Institut für Flugmedizin. Aktuelle Forschungsarbeiten aus dem Institut für Flugmedizin. Linder Höhe, Germany: Abteilung Wissenschaftliches Berichtswesen der Deutschen Forschungs, 1973.

Institute of Medicine, Division of Health Sciences Policy. Airline Pilot Age, Health and Performance. Washington, DC, USA: National Academy Press, 1981.

International Air Transport Association. Flight Crew Training. Montreal, Quebec, Canada: IATA, 1993.

International Air Transport Association. Human Factors in Aviation. Montreal, Quebec, Canada: IATA, 1994.

International Civil Aviation Organization. Human Factors in Air Traffic Control. Montreal, Canada: ICAO, 1993.

International Civil Aviation Organization. Operational Implications of Automation in Advanced Technology Flight Decks. Montreal, Canada: ICAO, 1992.

Isaac AR, Ruitenberg B. Air Traffic Control: Human Performance Factors. England – USA: Ashgate, 1999.

Jensen RS. Aviation Psychology. Brookfield, VT, USA: Gower Publishing Co., 1989.

Jensen RS. Pilot Judgment and Crew Resource Management. England – USA: Ashgate, 1995.

Johnston N, McDonald N. Aviation Psychology in Practice. England – USA: Ashgate, 1997.

Kern T. Controlling Pilot Error: Culture, Environment, and CRM. New York, NY, USA: McGraw-Hill, 2001.

Kern T. Darker Shades of Blue: The Rogue Pilot. New York, NY, USA: McGraw-Hill, 1999.

Kern T. Flight Discipline. New York, NY, USA: McGraw-Hill, 1998.

King RE. Aerospace Clinical Psychology. England – USA: Ashgate, 1999.

Kirchhoff HW. Stress und Fliegen Sowie Aktuelle Probleme der Flugmedizin. Darmstadt, Germany: Wehr und Wissen Verlagsgesellschaft, 1968.

Kovalenko PA. Aviameditsinskie I Ergonomicheskie Issiedovaniia Chelovecheskogo Faktora v Grazhdanskoi Aviatsii. Moskva, USSR: Gosudarstvennyi Nauchno, 1990.

Lareo JM. Factores Humanos en Aviación. Madrid, Spain: Iberia - Líneas Aéreas de España (publicación interna), 1989.

Leimann Patt HO. Psiquiatria Aeronáutica Sistémica. Buenos Aires, Argentina: Editorial Kargieman, 1987.

Maurino DE. Beyond Aviation Human Factors: Safety in High Technology Systems. England – USA: Ashgate, 1998.

McFarland RA. Human Factors in Air Transport Design. New York, NY, USA: McGraw-Hill Book Co., 1946.

McFarland RA. Human Factors in Air Transportation. New York, NY, USA: McGraw Hill Book Co., 1953.

McGann B. Psychological Aspects of Transmeridian Flying. Dublin, Ireland: Institute of Psychology, 1971.

McIntrye GR. Patterns in Safety Thinking: A Literature Guide to Air Transportation Safety. England – USA: Ashgate, 2000.

Meo E. Psicologia e Psicopatologia, Nozioni Applicate alla Medicina Aeronautica. Torino, Italy: I.T.E.R., 1940.

Miller JC. Controlling Pilot Error: Fatigue. New York, NY, USA: McGraw-Hill, 2001.

Mohler SR, Nichamin HD. Aircrew Workload. In Siegriest CJ, Wegmann HM. Breakdown in Human Adaptation to Stress. Vol. 1, Der Haag: M. Nighoff Publishers, 1984.

Mortimer RG, Hanson JS. Aviation Safety Research: Literature Review of Sources of Aviation Accident and Incident Data and Selected Factors Contributing to Accidents. Champaign, IL, USA: University of Illinois, 1993.

National Academy of Sciences, National Research Council, Space Science Board. Human Factors in Long-Duration Spaceflight. Washington, DC, USA: National Academy Press, 1972.

National Aeronautics and Space Administration. An Introduction to the Assurance of Human Performance in Space Systems. Washington, DC, USA: U.S. Government Printing Office, NASA Special Publication # 6506. 1968.

National Safety Council. Safety Handbook Aviation Ground Operation. Itasca, IL, USA: National Safety Council, 2000.

Nolan MS. Fundamentals of Air Traffic Control. Pacific Grove, CA, USA: Brooks/Cole, 1999.

Ocker WC, Crane CJ. Blind Flight in Theory and Practice. San Antonio, TX, USA: Naylor Printing Co., 1932.

O'Hare D. Human Performance in General Aviation. England – USA: Ashgate, 1999.

O'Hare D, Roscoe S. Flightdeck Performance - The Human Factor. USA: Iowa State University Press, 1990.

O'Neil HF, Andrews DH. Aircrew Training and Assessment. Mahwah, NJ, USA: Lawrence Erlbaum Associates Publishers, 2000.

Orlady HW, Orlady LM. Human Factors in Multi-Crew Flight Operations. England – USA: Ashgate, 1999.

Parry JB, Fokkema SD. Aviation Psychology in Western-Europe. Amsterdam, Netherlands: Swets & Seitlinger, 1958.

Platonov KK. Psikhologiia Letnogo Truda. Moskva, USSR: 1960.

Ponomarenko V, Boubel T. Kingdom in the Sky: Earthly Fetters and Heavenly Freedoms: The Pilot's Approach to the Military Flight Environment. Neuilly-sur-Seine, France: RTO/NATO, 2000.

Ponomarenko V, Zavalova N. Prakticheskaia Psikhologiia: Problemy Bezopasnosti Letnogo Truda. Moskva, Russia: Nauka, 1994.

Prew SJ. Survival for Aircrew. England – USA: Ashgate, 1999.

Reinhart RO. Human Factors in Pilot Performance. Blue Ridge Summit, PA, USA: TAB Books, 1991.

Richards W, Dismukes K. Vision Research for Flight Simulation. Washington, D. C., USA: National Academy Press, 1982.

Section III. Publications in Other Topics Related to Aerospace Medicine

Rohmert W. Becker-Biskaborn GU. Psycho-Physische Belastung und Beanspruchung von Fluglotsen. Stuttgart, Germany: Gentner, 1973.

Roscoe SN. Aviation Psychology. USA: The Iowa State University Press/NASA-AMES Research Center, 1980.

Roske-Hofstrand RJ, Murphy ED. Human Information Processing in Air Traffic Control. San Diego, CA, USA: Academic Press, 1998.

Sarter NB, Amalberti R. Cognitive Engineering in the Aviation Domain. Mahwah, NJ, USA: Erlbaum, 2000.

Seamster TL. Developing Advanced Crew Resource Management (ACRM) Training: A Training Manual. Washington, DC, USA: U.S. Department of Transportation, Federal Aviation Administration, 1998.

Seamster TL, Redding RE. Applied Cognitive Task Analysis in Aviation. England – USA: Avebury Aviation, 1997.

Sells SB, Berry CA. Human Factors in Jet and Space Travel - A Medical Psychological Analysis. New York, NY, USA: The Ronald Press Co., 1961.

Sidorov OA. Fiziologicheskie Faktory Cheloveka, Opredeliaiushchie Komponovku Posta Upravieniia Mashionoi. Moskva, USSR: 1962.

Smith GM, Dismukes K. Facilitation and Debriefing in Aviation Training and Operations. England – USA: Ashgate, 2000.

Smolensky MW, Stein ES. Human Factors in Air Traffic Control. San Diego, CA, USA: Academic Press, 1998.

Society of Automotive Engineers. Education, Training, and Human Engineering in Aerospace. Warrendale, PA, USA: Society of Automotive Engineers, 1993.

Southwest Research Institute. Final Report on Biotechnology Research Requirements for Aeronautical Systems Through the Year 2000, Volumes I and II. San Antonio, TX, USA: Air Force Office of Scientific Research, Contract Report F496-20-81-C-0059, 1982.

Stokes A, Kite K. Flight Stress: Stress, Fatigue, and Performance in Aviation. England – USA: Ashgate, 1994.

Strollo M. Psicologia Generale e Applicata all'Aeronautica. Firenze, Italy: Scuola de Guerra Aerea, 1959.

Stupakov GP, Syrovatko VG. Entsiklopedicheskii Spravochnik po Aviatsionnoi Ergonomike I Ekologii. Moskva, Russia: Izd-vo IP RAN, 1997.

Taylor RL. Human Factors: The Force Within. Greenwich, CT, USA: Belvoir Publications, 1991.

Telfer R. Aviation Instruction and Training. England – USA: Ashgate, 1993.

Telfer R, Moore PJ. Aviation Training: Learners, Instruction, and Organization. England – USA: Avebury Aviation, 1997.

Thomas M. Managing Pilot Stress. England – USA: MacMillan Publishing Company, 1989.

Transport Canada, Air Canada Human Factors Project Team. Human Factors for Aviation: Advanced Handbook. Ottawa, Canada: Transport Canada, 1996.

Transport Canada, Air Canada Human Factors Project Team. Human Factors for Aviation: Insturctor's Guide. Ottawa, Canada: Transport Canada, 1996.

Trollip SF, Jensen, RS. Human Factors for General Aviation. Englewood, CO, USA: Jeppesen Sanderson, 1991.

Turner TP. Cockpit Resource Management: The Private Pilot's Guide. New York NY, USA: TAB Books, 1995.

Umanskii SP. Bar'er Vynoslivosti Letchika. Moskva, USSR: Mashinostroenie, 1964.

U.S. Department of the Navy, Bureau of Aeronautics. The Effects of Flight: Physical and Mental Aspects. New York - London: McGraw-Hill Book Co., Inc., 1943.

Varney A. The Psychology of Flight. Toronto - New York - London: D. Van Nostrand Co. Inc., 1950.

Weiner EL, Kanki BG. Cockpit Resource Management. San Diego, CA, USA: Academic Press, 1993.

Weiner EL, Nagel DC. Human Factors in Aviation. San Diego - New York - Boston: Academic Press, Inc., 1988.

Wickens CD. The Future of Air Traffic Control: Human Operators and Automation. Washington, DC, USA: National Academy Press, 1998.

Wickens CD, Mavor AS. Flight to the Future: Human Factors in Air Traffic Control. Washington, DC, USA: National Academy Press, 1997.

Wiggins MW, Stevens C. Aviation Social Science: Research Methods in Practice. England – USA: Ashgate, 1999.

Wise JA, Hopkin VD. Automation and Systems Issues in Air Traffic Control. Germany – USA: Springer-Verlag, 1991.

Wise JA, Hopkin VD. Human Factors in Certification. Mahwah, NJ, USA: Lawrence Erlbaum Associates Publishers, 2000.

Wise JA, Hopkin VD. Verification and Validation of Complex Systems: Additional Human Factors Issues. Daytona Beach, FL, USA: Embry-Riddle Aeronautical University Press, 1993.

Wood RH. Aviation Safety Programs: A Management Handbook. Englewood, CO, USA: Jeppesen Sanderson, 1997.

Zeier H. Psychophysiologiche Stressforschung: Methodik und Ergebnisse einer Untersuchung bei Flugverkehrsleitern. Bern, Switzerland: Verlag Paul Haupt, 1992.

General Human Factors and Psychology

Akerstedt T. Wide Awake at Odd Hours: Shift Work, Time Zones and Burning the Midnight Oil. Stockholm, Sweden: Swedish Council for Work Life Research, 1996.

Andreassi JL. Psychophysiology: Human Behavior and Physiological Response. Mahwah, NJ, USA: Lawrence Erlbaum Associates, 2000.

Androile SJ, Adelman L. Cognitive Systems Engineering for User-Computer Interface Design, Prototyping, and Evaluation. Hillsdale, NJ, USA: Lawrence Erlbaum Associates, 1995.

Applezweig MH. Psychological Stress and Related Concepts. New London, CT, USA: Connecticut College for Women, 1957.

Beehr TA. Psychological Stress in the Workplace. England – USA: Routledge, 1994.

Boff KR, Kaufman L, Thomas JP. Handbook of Perception and Human Performance. Vol. II, New York, NY, USA: Wiley, 1986.

Chapanis A. Human Factors in Systems Engineering. New York, NY, USA: Wiley, 1996.

Clark WG, Del Giudice J. Principles of Psychopharmacology. New York, NY, USA: Academic Press, 1978.

Clegg S, Hardy C. Handbook of Organization Studies. England – USA: Sage Publications, 1996.

Davis DR, Parasuraman R. The Psychology of Vigilance. London, England: Academic Press, 1981.

Dikaia LG, Zankovskii AN. Psikhologicheskie Problemy Professional'noi Deiatel'nosti. Moskva, Russia: Nauka, 1991.

Driskell JE, Salas E. Stress and Human Performance. Mahwah, NJ, USA: Lawrence Erlbaum Associates, 1996.

Fisher JD, Bell PA, Baum A. Environmental Psychology. New York, NY, USA: Holt, Rinehart & Winston, 1984.

Fisk AD, Rogers WA. Handbook of Human Factors and the Older Adult. San Diego, CA, USA: Academic Press, 1997.

Fitts PM, Posner MI. Human Performance. Westport, USA: Greenwood Press, 1967.

Flach J. Global Perspectives on the Ecology of Human-Machine Systems. Hillsdale, NJ, USA: Lawrence Erlbaum Associates Publishers, 1995.

Flin RH. Decision Making Under Stress: Emerging Themes and Applications. England – USA: Ashgate, 1997.

Frolov, MV. Funktsional'noe Sostoianie Cheloveka I Metody ego Issiedovaniia: Sbornik Nauchnykh Turdov. Moskva, Russia: Nauka, 1992.

Gaillard JP. Psychologie de l'Homme au Travail: les Relations Homme-Machine. Paris, France: Dunod, 1997.

Gawron VJ. Human Performance Measures Handbook. Mahwah, NJ, USA: Lawrence Erlbaum Associates, 2000.

Gilmore WE, Gertman D. The User-Computer Interface in Process Control: A Human Factors Engineering Handbook. Boston, MA, USA: Academic Press, 1989.

Hancock PA. Human Factors Psychology. Amsterdam, Holland: North Holland, 1987.

Hancock PA. Human Performance and Ergonomics. San Diego, CA, USA: Academic Press, 1999.

Hancock PA, Desmond PA. Stress, Workload, and Fatigue. Mahwah, NJ, USA: Lawrence Erlbaum Associates Publishers, 2001.

Hancock PA., and Meshkati. Human Mental Workload. Amsterdam, Holland: North Holland, 1988.

Holahan CJ. Environmental Psychology. New York, NY, USA: Random House, 1982.

Holding DH. Human Skills - Studies in Human Performance. Chichester: John Wiley & Sons, 1981.

Hollnagel E. Human Reliability Analysis: Context and Control. England – USA: Academic Press, 1993.

Huchingson RD. New Horizons for Human Factors in Design. New York, NY, USA: McGraw-Hill Book Company, 1981.

Section III. Publications in Other Topics Related to Aerospace Medicine

Jones DM, Smith AP. Handbook of Human Performance. England – USA: Academic Press, 1992.

Jordan PW. An Introduction to Usability. England – USA: Taylor & Francis, 1998.

Kahneman D. Attention and Effort. Englewood Cliffs, NJ, USA: Prentice-Hall, 1973.

Kantowitz BH, Roediger HL. Experimental Psychology. St. Paul, MN, USA: West Publishing, 1984.

Kantowitz BH, Sorkin RD. Human Factors: Understanding People-System Relationships. New York, NY, USA: Wiley, 1983.

Kline P. The Handbook of Psychological Testing. England – USA: Routledge, 1993.

Kroemer KHE, Grandjean E. Fitting the Task to the Human: A Textbook of Occupational Ergonomics. England – USA: Taylor & Francis, 1997.

Kroemer KHE, Kroemer HJ. Engineering Physiology: Bases of Human Factors/Ergonomics. New York, NY, USA: Van Nostrand Reinhold, 1997.

Kroemer KHE, Kroemer HJ, Kroemer-Elbert KF. Engineering Physiology: Bases of Human Factors/ Ergonomics. Florence, KY, USA: Van Nostrand Reinhold, 1990.

Kvalseth TO. Ergonomics of Workstation Design. London, England: Butterworths, 1983.

Leach J. Survival Psychology. Washington Square, NY, USA: New York University Press, 1994.

Leplat J. Regards sur l'Activité en Situation de Travail: Contribution à la Psychologie Ergonomique. Paris, France: Presses Universitaires de France, 1997.

Luce GG. Biological Rhythms in Psychiatry and Medicine. Rockville, MD, USA: U.S. National Institute of Mental Health, 1978.

Maier NR, Verser GC. Psychology in Industrial Organizations. Boston, MA, USA: Houghton Mifflin Company, 1982.

Matthews G. Human Performance: Cognition, Stress, and Individual Differences. England – USA: Taylor & Francis, 2000.

McCormick EJ, Sanders M. Human Factors in Engineering and Design. New York, NY, USA: McGraw-Hill, 1982.

Meister D. The History of Human Factors and Ergonomics. Mahwah, NJ, USA: Lawrence Erlbaum Associates, 1999.

Meister D. Human Factors - Theory and Practice. New York, NY, USA: John Wiley & Sons, 1971.

Meister D. Psychology of System Design. Netherlands – England: Elsevier, 1991.

Meister D, Rabideau GF. Human Factors Evaluation in System Development. New York, NY, USA: John Wiley & Sons, 1965.

Monk TH. Sleep, Sleepiness, and Performance. England – USA: Wiley, 1991.

Monk TH, Folkard S. Making Shift Work Tolerable. London, England: Taylor & Francis, 1992.

Moray N. Mental Workload - Its Theory and Measurement. New York, NY, USA: Plenum, 1979.

Morgan CT, Cook JS, Chapanis A, Lund MW. Human Engineering Guide to Equipment Design. New York, NY, USA: McGraw-Hill, 1963.

Mouloua M, Koonce JM. Human-Automation Interaction: Research and Practice. Mahwah, NJ, USA: Lawrence Erlbaum Associates, 1997.

Nielsen J. Usability Engineering. San Francisco, CA, USA: Morgan Kaufmann Publishers, 1994.

O'Brien, TG, Charlton SG. Handbook of Human Factors Testing and Evaluation. Mahwah, NJ, USA: Lawrence Erlbaum Associates, 1996.

Parasuraman R, Mouloua M. Automation and Human Performance: Theory and Applications. Mahwah, NJ, USA: Lawrence Erlbaum Associates, 1996.

Parsons HM. Man-Machine System Experiments. Baltimore, MD, USA: Johns Hopkins Press, 1972.

Perrow C. Normal Accidents: Living with High-Risk Technologies: With a New Afterword and a Postscript on the Y2K Problem. Princeton, NJ, USA: Princeton University Press, 1999.

Pick HW, Leibowitz JE, Singer JE, Steinschneiden A, Stevenson HW. Psychology - From Research to Practice. New York, NY, USA: Plenum Press, 1978.

Poulton EC. Environment and Human Efficiency. Springfield, IL, USA: Charles C. Thomas, 1970.

Poulton EC. Tracking Skill and Manual Control. New York, NY, USA: Academic Press, Inc., 1974.

Powell DH, Whitla DK. Profiles in Cognitive Aging. Cambridge, MA, USA: Harvard University Press, 1994.

Proctor RW, Van Zandt T. Human Factors in Simple and Complex Systems. Boston, MA, USA: Allyn and Bacon, 1994.

Reason JT. Human Error. Cambridge, England: Cambridge University Press, 1990.

Reason JT. Managing the Risks of Organizational Accidents. England – USA: Ashgate, 1997.

Robinson JO. The Psychology of Visual Illusion. London, England: Hutchinson, 1972.

Roscoe SN, Cori L. Predicting Human Performance. Pierrefonds, Quebec, Canada: Helio Press, 1997.

Salvendy G. Handbook of Human Factors and Ergonomics. New York, NY, USA: Wiley, 1997.

Salvendy G, Seymour WD. Prediction and Development of Industrial Work Performance. New York, NY, USA: Wiley, 1973.

Sanders MS, McCormick EJ. Human Factors in Engineering and Design. New York, NY, USA: McGraw-Hill, 1993.

Satchell PM. Innovation and Automation. England – USA: Ashgate, 1998.

Scerbo MW, Mouloua M. Automation Technology and Human Performance: Current Research and Trends. Mahwah, NJ, USA: Lawrence Erlbaum Associates, 1999.

Scholz RW, Zimmer AC. Qualitative Aspects of Decision Making. Lengerich, Germany: Pabst Science Publishers, 1997.

Senders JW, Moray N. Human Error: Cause, Prediction, and Reduction. Hillsdale, NJ, USA: Lawrence Erlbaum Associates Publishers, 1991.

Stanford SC, Salmon P. Stress: From Synapse to Syndrome. San Diego, CA, USA: Academic Press, 1993.

Stanton N, Young MA. A Guide to Methodology in Ergonomics: Designing for Human Use. England – USA: Taylor & Francis, 1999.

Stevens S. Handbook of Experimental Psychology. New York, NY, USA: John Wiley & Sons, 1951.

Stokois D, Altman I. Handbook of Environmental Psychology. Malabar, FL, USA: Krieger Publishing Company, 1991.

Stolovitch HD, Keeps EJ. Handbook of Human Performance Technology: Improving Individual and Organizational Performance Worldwide. San Francisco, CA, USA: Jossey-Bass/Pfeiffer, 1999.

Svenson O, Maule AJ. Time Pressure and Stress in Human Judgment and Decision Making. New York: Plenum Press, 1993.

Troland LT. A Handbook of General Experimental Psychology. Worcester, England: Clark University Press, 1934.

Van Cott HP, Kinkade RG. Human Engineering Guide to Equipment Design. Washington, DC, USA: U. S. Government Printing Office, 1972.

Venda VF, Venda YV. Dynamics in Ergonomics, Psychology, and Decisions: Introduction to Ergodynamics. Norwood, NJ, USA: Ablex Publishing Corporation, 1995.

Warm J. Sustained Attention in Human Performance. London, England: Wiley, 1984.

Welch B, Welch AS. Psychological Effects of Noise. New York, NY, USA: Plenum Press, 1970.

Wexley KN, Yuki GA. Organizational Behavior and Industrial Psychology: Readings with Commentary. New York, NY, USA: Oxford University Press, 1975.

Wickens CD. Engineering Psychology and Human Performance. Columbus, OH, USA: Merrill, 1984.

Wickens CD, Hollands JG. Engineering Psychology and Human Performance. Upper Saddie River, NJ, USA: Prentice Hall, 2000.

Wilson JR, Corlett EN. Evaluation of Human Work: A Practical Ergonomics Methodology. Bristol, PA, USA: Taylor & Francis, 1995.

Zinchenko VP, Leonova AB. The Psychometrics of Fatigue (translated from the Russian). England – USA: Taylor & Francis, 1985.

Aerospace Medicine History

Aerospace Medical Association. Sixty Years of Aerospace Medicine: Index to *Aviation, Space, and Environmental Medicine* v. 1-60. Alexandria, VA, USA: AsMA, 1995.

Andreotti G. Padre Gemelli e la Medicina Aeronautica. Milano, Italy: Vita e Pensiero, 1965.

Babiichuk AN. Chelovek, Nebo, Kosmos. Moskva, USSR: Voenizdat, 1979.

Baker D. The History of Manned Space Flight. New York, NY, USA: Crown Publishers, 1981.

Beaven CL. A Chronological History of Aviation Medicine. Flight Surg. Top., 1938; 2(4):185-206.

Benford RJ. The Heritage of Aviation Medicine - An Annotated Directory of Early Artifacts. Washington, DC, USA: Aerospace Medical Association, 1979.

Bochenkov AA. Iz Istorii Razvitiia Otechestvennoi Aviatsionnoi I Kosmicheskoi Meditsiny. Leningrad, USSR: Nauch, 1989.

Byrom J. Fields of Air: Triumphs, Tragedies, and Mysteries of Civil Aviation in Southern Africa. Rivonia South Africa: Ashanti Publishing, 1993.

Section III. Publications in Other Topics Related to Aerospace Medicine

Canaveris G. The History of Aviation Medicine in Argentina. Aviat. Space and Environ. Med. 1990; 61:955-61.

Carlson ET, Heveran BT. Benjamin Rush and the Birth of American Aviation Medicine. Aerospace Medicine 1974; 45:1083.

Charlet R. Les Medecins Francais et L'aeronautique. Pr. Med., 1935; 43:1373-1374.

Cuppers S. Die Geschichtliche Entwicklung der Höhenphysiologie und ihre Bedeutung für die Luftfahrtmedizin bis 1961. Aachen, Germany: Verlag Shaker, 1994.

Davis WR. The Development of Aviation Medicine. Milit. Surg., 1923; 53:207-217.

Dempsey CA. 50 Years of Research on Man in Flight. Dayton, OH, USA: Air Force Aerospace Medical Research Laboratory, Wright Patterson AFB, 1985.

Garsaux PA. Histoire Anecdotique de la Medicine de L'Air. Paris, France: Editions Du Scorpion, 1963.

Gemelli A. Padre Gemelli e la Medicina Aeronautica. Milano, Italy: Editrice Vita e Pensiero, 1965.

Gibson TM., Harrison MH. Into Thin Air - A History of Aviation Medicine in the RAF. London, England: R. Hale, 1984.

Gomez-Cabezas P. La Medicina Aeronáutica desde sus Orígenes hasta la Era Aeronáutica. Madrid, Spain: Instituto de Historia y Cultura Aeronáutica, 1987.

Gowdey DW, Pearce JW. A Selected Bibliography of the Open Literature on Aviation Medicine, 1945-1955. Ottawa, Canada: Defence Research Board, 1955.

Herlitzka A. L'Opera del Medico per il Progresso dell'Aviazione. Int. Air. Congr. (Rome), 1927; 4:568-581.

Hitchcock FA. Paul Bert and the Beginnings of Aviation Medicine. Aerosp. Med., 1971; 42(10):1101-1107.

Hoff EC, Fulton JF. A Bibliography of Aviation Medicine. Illinois - Maryland, USA: Charles C. Thomas, 1942.

Hoff PM, Hoff EC. A Bibliography of Aviation Medicine: Supplement. Washington, DC, USA: National Research Council, 1944.

Hoffman MA. Ross A. MacFarland Collection in Aerospace Medicine and Human Factors Engineering. Dayton, OH, USA: Fordham Health Sciences Library, Wright State University School of Medicine, 1987.

Hough MM. United States Army Air Ambulance: Concise Histories and Lineages of Army Aeromedical Units from the Korean War to the Present. Bellevue, WA, USA: Vedder River Publishing Company, 1999.

Houston CS. Going High, the Story of Man and Altitude. New York, NY, USA: American Alpine Club, 1980.

Hume EE. Colonel Robert Picque, a Pioneer in Aviation Medicine. Milit. Surg. 1929; 65:612-614.

Iriarte DR. Historia de la Medicina Aeronáutica en Venezuela. Caracas, Venezuela: 1985.

Kerr WK. Bibliography of Canadian Reports in Aviation Medicine, 1939-1945. Ottawa, Canada: Defence Research Board, 1962.

Lauschner EA. The Beginnings of Aviation Medicine in Germany. Aviat. Space & Environ. Med. **XXX**, 1984.

Munn NL. An Historical Introduction to Aviation Psychology. Washington, DC, USA: Civil Aeronautics Administration, 1942.

Neel SH, Shamburek RH. History of Army Aviation Medicine. U. S. Army Aviation Digest, 1963; 9(1):17.

Neuberger JF. Aviation Medicine in the United States Navy. Nav. Med. Bull., 1922; 16:834-844.

Nicholson AN. Neurosciences and Aviation Medicine: A Century of Endeavour. New Zealand: International Academy of Aviation and Space Medicine, 1998.

Novikov VS. Istoriia Kafedry Aviatsionnoi I Kosmicheskoi Meditsiny: K 200-Letiiu Voenno-Meditsinskoi Akademii. Sankt-Peterburg, Russia: Nauka, 1995.

Peyton G. 50 Years of Aerospace Medicine - 1918 to 1968. Washington DC, USA: AFSC Historical Publications, Series No. 67-180, 1967.

Platonov KK. Istorii Otechestvennoi Aviatsionnoi Psikhologii: Dokumenty I Materialy. Moskva, USSR: Meditsina, 1981.

Püschel E. Die Seenotverbände der Deutschen Luftwaffe und ihr Sanitätsdienst 1939-1945: Aufgaben, Leistungen, Probleme. Düsseldorf, Germany: Droste, 1978.

Robinson DH. The Dangerous Sky: A History of Aviation Medicine. Seattle, WA, USA: University of Washington Press, 1973.

Sergeev AA. Ocherki po Istorii Aviatsionnoi Meditsiny. Moskva, USSR: Akademii Navk 1962.

Tredici TH. Aerospace Ophthalmology: History an Review. San Antonio, TX, USA: USAF School of Aerospace Medicine, Brooks AFB, 1986.

Tuliakov MI. Baikonur, Kosmos, Zdorov'e. Baikonur, Kazakhstan: Space Center, 1995.

Tuttle AD, Armstrong HG. The Role of Aviation Medicine in the Development of Aviation. Milit. Surg. 1939; 85:285-301.

West JB. High Life: A History of High-Altitude Physiology and Medicine. New York, NY, USA: Oxford University Press, 1998.

White WJ. A History of the Centrifuge in Aerospace Medicine. Santa Monica, CA, USA: Douglas Aircraft Corporation, 1964.

Wilmer WH. The Early Development of Aviation Medicine in the United States. Milit. Surg. 1935; 77:115-135.

Zebouni FH. Forty Years of Aviation Medicine 1951-1991. Beirut, Lebanon: Middle East Airlines Medical Department, 1991.

IV) PROCEEDINGS FROM SCIENTIFIC MEETINGS IN AEROSPACE MEDICINE AND PSYCHOLOGY

Aero Medical Association. Congres Mondial de Medicine Aeronautique - 3e Congres Europeen. Bruxelles, Belgium: Impr. de la Barriere. 1958.

Aero Medical Association. Deuxieme Congress de la Branche D' Expression Francaise. Bruxelles, Belgium. 1954.

Aerospace Medical Association. Proceedings of the Annual Scientific Meetings (1929-1990). 320 South Henry St., Alexandria, VA 22314-3524, USA.

Aviation Medicine Symposium. Toxic Hazards in Military Flying and in the Aviation Industry: Aviation Medicine Symposium held at the Headquarters Air Material Command, 1957. Wright-Patterson Air Force Base, OH, USA: 1957.

Bedwell T, Strughold H. Bioastronautics and the Exploration of Space: The Proceedings of the Third International Symposium. San Antonio, TX, USA: U.S. Air Force Systems Command, 1965.

Bier V. Proceedings of Workshop on Accident Sequence Precursors and Probabilistic Risk Analysis: Madison, Wisconsin, USA, 1995. College Park, MD, USA: Center for Reliability Engineering, 1998.

Busby DE. Recent Advances in Aerospace Medicine - 18th International Congress of Aviation and Space Medicine. Reidel Dordrecht Publishing Co., New York, USA. 1970.

Commission of the European Communities. Cosmic Radiation and Aircrew Exposure: Implementation of European Requirements in Civil Aviation: Proceedings of an International Conference, Dublin, Ireland, July 1-3, 1998. Ashford, Kent, England: Nuclear Technology Publishing, 1999.

Commission of the European Communities. Radiation Exposure of Civil Aircrew: Proceedings of a Workshop in Luxembourg, June 25-27, 1991. Ashford, Kent, England: Nuclear Technology Publishing, 1993.

Congrès International de l'Aviation Sanitaire. Premier Congrès. Paris, France: Tancrède, 1929.

Congrès Mondial de Médecine Aéronautique: 3e Congrès Européen. Louvain, Belgium: 1958.

II Congreso Mondiale di Medicina Aeronautica e Spaziale (IV Congreso Aeropeo di Medicina Aeronautica e Spaziale. Tipografía del Senato Del Dott. G. Bardi, Rome, Italy. 1961.

V Congresso di Medicina Aeronautica. Napoli, Rome: Tipografía Regionale. 1953.

VI Congresso Internazionale e XII Europeo de Medicina Aeronautica e Spaziale. Rome, Italy: 1964.

Draeger J, Schwartz R. Forty-First International Congress of Aviation and Space Medicine: 12-16 September 1993, Hamburg. Bologna, Italy: Moduzzi Editore, International Proceedings Division, 1994.

European Undersea Biomedical Society. Proceedings of the Annual Meeting of the European Undersea Biomedical Society: 1981 – current.

Federation of American Societies for Experimental Biology. Symposium on Underwater Physiology: Proceedings 1972-1975. Bethesda, MD, USA: FASEB, 1976 and 1978.

Gilson RD, Garland DJ. Situational Awareness in Complex Systems: Proceedings of a CAHFA Conference. Daytona Beach, FL, USA: Embry-Riddle Aeronautical University Press, 1994.

Hannisdahl B, Sem-Jacobsen CW. Aviation and Space Medicine: Proceedings of the International Congress of Aviation and Space Medicine, Oslo. Oslo, Norway: Universitestforlaget, 1969.

Section IV. *Proceedings From Scientific Meetings in Aerospace Medicine and Psychology*

Harma M. New Challenges for the Organization of Night and Shift Work: Proceedings of the XIII International Symposium on Night and Shift Work: June 1997, Finland. Helsinki, Finland: Finnish Institute of Occupational Health, 1998.

Harris D. Transportation Systems, Medical Ergonomics and Training. Second International Conference on Engineering Psychology and Cognitive Ergonomics, Oxford, England, 1998. England: Ashgate, 1999.

Hartley L. Managing Fatigue in Transportation: Proceedings of the 3rd Fatigue in Transportation Conference, Fremantle, Western Australia, 1998. New York, NY, USA: Pergamon, 1998.

Hayward BJ, Lowe AR. Applied Aviation Psychology: Achievement, Change, and Challenge: Proceedings of the Third Australian Aviation Psychology Symposium. England – USA: Avebury Aviation, 1996.

European Congress of Aviation Medicine, 4th. Rome, Italy, 1959.

I European Congress of Aviation Medicine. Scheveningen, Hague: Soesterberg. 1956.

International Academy of Aviation and Space Medicine, Proceedings of the Annual Scientific Meetings (1953-1990) Lisbon Airport, P. O. Box 5194, 1704 Lisbon Codex, Portugal.

Internetional Civil Aviation Organization. Proceedings of the Third ICAO Global Flight Safety and Human Factors Symposium: Auckland, Australia, April 1996. Montreal, Canada: International Civil Aviation Organization, 1996.

International Civil Aviation Organization. Proceedings of the Fourth ICAO Global Flight Safety and Human Factors Symposium: Santiago, Chile, April 1999. Montreal, Canada: International Civil Aviation Organization, 1999.

International Symposium on Basic Environmental Problems of Man in Space. Proceedings 1-6. International Astronautical Federation – International Academy of Astronautics. Austria – USA: Springer, 1962-1980.

Jensen RS. Proceedings of the International Symposium on Aviation Psychology: 1st – 10th. Columbus, OH, USA: Ohio State University, Aviation Psychology Laboratory, 1981 – 1999.

Johnston N, Fuller R. Proceedings of the 21st Conference of the European Association for Aviation Psychology: v. 1 Applications of Psychology to the Aviation System; v. 2 Aviation Psychology Training and Selection; v. 3 Human Factors in Aviation Operations. England – USA: Ashgate, 1995.

Lamb LE. The First International Symposium on Cardiology in Aviation. USAF School of Aviation Medicine, Brooks AFB - USAF Aerospace Medical Center, San Antonio, Texas, USA. 1959.

Lowe AR, Hayward BJ. Aviation Resource Management: Proceedings of the Fourth Australian Aviation Psychology Symposium. Manly, Australia: Ashgate, 2000.

Musacchia XJ, Jansky L. Survival in the Cold: Hibernation and Other Adaptations: Proceedings of the International Symposium for Survival in the Cold. New York, NY, USA: Elsevier, 1981.

National Academy of Sciences - National Research Council. Impact Acceleration Stress: With a Comprehensive Chronological Bibliography. USAF School of Aviation Medicine, Brooks AFB, Nov. 27-29, 1962.

National Aeronautics and Space Administration. Twelfth Man in Space Symposium: The Future of Humans in Space, June 8-13, 1997, Washington, DC. France – USA, 1997.

National Aeronautics and Space Administration - Universities Space Research Association - Baylor College of Medicine - International Academy of Astronautics. Physiologic Adaptation of Man in Space: 7th International Man in Space Symposium. Houston, TX, U.S.A. 1986.

National Luchtvaartgeneeskundig Centrum. Premier Congress Europeen de Medicine Aeronautique. Soesterberg, Netherlands. 1957.

National Research Council – Panel on Underwater Swimmers. Proceedings of the Underwater Physiology Symposium. Washington, DC, USA: National Academy of Sciences, 1955-1971.

North Atlantic Treaty Organization – Advisory Group for Aerospace Research and Development – Aerospace Medical Panel Symposium. Aeromedical Support Issues in Contingency Operations. Rotterdam, Netherlands, 1997.

North Atlantic Treaty Organization – Advisory Group for Aerospace Research and Development – Aerospace Medical Panel Symposium. Aircraft Accidents: Trends in Aerospace Medicine Investigation Techniques. Cesme, Turkey, 1992.

North Atlantic Treaty Organization – Advisory Group for Aerospace Research and Development – Aerospace Medical Panel Symposium. Allergic, Immunological and Infectious Disease Problems in Aerospace Medicine. Rome, Italy, 1991.

North Atlantic Treaty Organization – Advisory Group for Aerospace Research and Development – Aerospace Medical Panel Symposium. The Clinical Basis for Aeromedical Decision Making. Palma de Mallorca, Spain, 1994.

North Atlantic Treaty Organization – Advisory Group for Aerospace Research and Development – Aerospace Medical Panel Symposium. Neurological Limitations of Aircraft Operations: Human Performance Implication. Cologne, Germany, 1995.

North Atlantic Treaty Organization – Advisory Group for Aerospace Research and Development – Aerospace Medical Panel Symposium. Selection and Training Advances in Aviation. Prague, Czech Republic, 1996.

North Atlantic Treaty Organization – Advisory Group for Aerospace Research and Development – Aerospace Medical Panel Symposium. Situation Awareness: Limitations and Enhancement in the Aviation Environment. Brussels, Belgium, 1995.

North Atlantic Treaty Organization – Research and Technology Organization - Human Factors and Medicine Panel Workshop. Aeromedical Aspects of Aircrew Training. San Diego, CA, USA, 1998.

North Atlantic Treaty Organization – Research and Technology Organization – Human Factors and Medicine Panel Workshop. Models for Aircrew Safety Assessment: Uses, Limitations and Requirements. Wright-Patterson Air Force Base, OH, USA, 1999.

North Atlantic Treaty Organization – Research and Technology Organization – Human Factors and Medicine Panel. Current Aeromedical Issues in Rotary Wing Operations. San Diego, CA, USA, 1998.

Roadman CH, Strughold H. Bioastronautics and the Exploration of Space: Proceedings of the Fourth International Symposium. Brooks Air Force Base, TX, USA: Aerospace Medical Division, 1968.

Royal Aeronautical Society. Human Factors for Aerospace Leaders: Proceedings, May 1996. London, England: Royal Aeronautical Society, 1996.

Soekkha HM. Aviation Safety: Human Factors, System Engineering, Flight Operations, Economics, Strategies, Management. Internetional Aviation Safety Conference, Rotterdam, Netherlands, 1997.

Specialists' Meeting on Models for Aircrew Safety Assessment. Models for Aircrew Safety Assessment: Uses, Limitations and Requirements. Neuilly-sur-Seine, France: NATO/RTO, 1999.

Symposium on Underwater Physiology. Underwater Physiology: Proceedings, 1955 – current.

Undersea Medical Society. Symposium on Underwater Physiology: Proceedings, 1978 and 1984. Bethesda, MD, USA: 1981 and 1984.

White CS, Benson OO. Physics and Medicine of the Upper Atmosphere - A Study of the Aeropause: Proceedings of a Symposium on the Physics and Medicine of the Upper Atmosphere. University of New Mexico Press, Albuquerque, New Mexico, USA. 1952.

Wise JA, Hopkin VD. Human Factors Certification of Advanced Aviation Technologies Conference (1993: Chateau de Bonas, France). Daytona Beach, FL, USA: Embry-Riddle Aeronautical University Press, 1994.

V) JOURNALS, NEWSLETTERS, AND BULLETINS IN AEROSPACE MEDICINE AND AEROSPACE HUMAN FACTORS

Acta Aerophysiologica. 1933-1934. Broschek & Company. Hamburg, Germany. (INACTIVE).

Advances in Space Biology and Medicine. JAI Press. Greenwich, CT, USA. (ACTIVE).

Advances in Space Research. Pergamon. England – USA. (ACTIVE).

Aeromedical & Training Digest. Environmental Tectonics Corporation. Southampton, PA, USA. (ACTIVE).

AeroMedical Journal. 1986-1992. 674 Via de la Valle, Suite 200, Solana Beach, CA, USA. (INACTIVE).

Aeromedical Reports. USAF School of Aerospace Medicine. Brooks Air Force Base, Texas, USA. (ACTIVE).

Aeromedical Review. USAF School of Aerospace Medicine. Brooks Air Force Base, TX, USA. (ACTIVE).

Aerospace Medicine. 1959-1974. Aerospace Medical Association. Washington, DC, USA. (INACTIVE).

Section V. Journals, Newsletters, and Bulletins in Aerospace Medicine and Aerospace Human Factors

Aerospace Medicine and Biology. NASA Scientific and Technical Information Facility. Baltimore, MD, USA. (ACTIVE).

Air Safety Week. PBI Media, LLC. Potomac, MD, USA. (ACTIVE).

Air Surgeons Bulletin. 1944-1945. U.S. Government Printing Office. Washington, DC, USA. (INACTIVE).

AirMed. Jems Communications. Carlsbad, CA, USA. (ACTIVE).

ASRS Directline. National Aeronautics and Space Administration. http://olias.arc.nasa.gov/asrs. (ACTIVE).

Aviakosmicheskaia I Ekologicheskaia Meditsina. Institut Mediko-Biologicheskikh Problem. Moskva, Russia. (ACTIVE).

Aviation Medicine. Aero Medical Society of India. Bangalore, India. (ACTIVE).

Aviation Medicine Quarterly. 1987-1991. Association of Aviation Medical Examiners of England, Wales and Northern Ireland. Wilmslow, Cheshire, U.K. (INACTIVE).

Aviation Safety. Belvoir Publications, Greenwich, CT, USA. (ACTIVE).

Aviation Safety Journal. 1991-1993. Federal Aviation Administration Office of the Assistant Administrator for Aviation Safety. Washington, DC, USA. (INACTIVE).

Aviation Safety Statistical Handbook. Federal Aviation Administration Air Traffic Resource Management Program. Washington, DC, USA. (ACTIVE).

Aviation, Space, and Environmental Medicine. Aerospace Medical Association. Alexandria, VA, USA. (ACTIVE).

Bulletin of the Iberoamerican Association of Aerospace Medicine. San Antonio, TX, USA. (ACTIVE).

Cabin Safety. The Write Partnership Limited. Hampshire, UK. (ACTIVE).

Contact. 1941-1959. U.S. Naval School of Aviation Medicine. Naval Air Station, Pensacola, Florida, USA. (INACTIVE).

Federal Air Surgeon's Medical Bulletin. Federal Aviation Administration Civil Aerospace Medical Institute. Oklahoma City, OK, USA. http://www. cami.jccbi.gov/aam-400A/fasmb.html. (ACTIVE).

Flight Surgeon Topics. 1937-1939. School of Aviation Medicine, Randolph Field. San Antonio, TX, USA. (INACTIVE).

Flightlines. Society of USAF Flight Surgeons. Brooks Air Force Base, TX, USA. (ACTIVE).

Flug-und Reisemedizin. Deutsche Gesellschaft fur Luft-und Raumfahrt-Medizin. Bonn, Germany. (ACTIVE).

Flying Safety. U.S. Air Force. Kirtland AFB, NM, USA (ACTIVE).

Gateway. Human Systems Information Analysis Center. Wright-Patterson AFB, OH, USA. http://iac.dtic.mil/hsiac. (ACTIVE).

Hang Tian yi Xue yu yi Xue Gong Cheng. Bejing, China. (ACTIVE).

Hanggong Uju Uihak. Han'guk Hanggong Uju Uihak Hyophoe. Seoul, Korea. (ACTIVE).

Hospital Aviation. 1982-1989. Aviation/Hospital Consultants. Orem, Utah, USA. (INACTIVE).

Human Factors and Aerospace Safety: An International Journal. Ashgate. England – USA. (ACTIVE).

Human Factors and Aviation Medicine. Flight Safety Foundation. Arlington, VA, USA. (ACTIVE).

International Aerospace Abstracts. American Institute of Aeronautics and Astronautics. New York, NY, USA. (ACTIVE).

International Journal of Aviation Psychology. Lawrence Erlbaum Associates Publishers. Hillsdale, NJ, USA. (ACTIVE).

Internationale Zeitschrift fur Angewandte Physiologie Einschliesslich Arbeitsphysiologie. 1955-1973. Springer-Verlag. Berlin, Germany. (INACTIVE).

ISASI Forum. International Society of Air Safety Investigators. Sterling, VA, USA. (ACTIVE).

Journal of Aero Medical Society of India. Institute of Aviation Medicine. 1967-1974. Bangalore, India. (INACTIVE).

Journal of Air Law and Commerce. Southern Methodist University School of Law. Dallas, TX, USA. (ACTIVE).

Journal of Aviation Medicine. 1930-1958. Aero Medical Association. Washington, DC, USA. (INACTIVE).

Journal of Human Performance in Extreme Environments. Society for Human Performance in Extreme Environments. League City, TX, USA. (ACTIVE).

Journal of Professional Aviation Training. Avex Ltd. Bath, United Kingdom. (ACTIVE).

Koku Igaku Jikkentai Hokoku. Koko Igaku Jikkentai. Tokyo, Japan. (ACTIVE).

Kosmicheskaia Biologiia I Aviakosmicheskaia Meditsina. Ministerstvo Zdravookhraneniia. 1974-1991. Moskva, USSR. (INACTIVE).

Kosmicheskaia Biologiia I Meditsina. Ministerstvo Zdravookharaneniia. 1967-1973. Moskva, USSR. (INACTIVE).

Life Sciences and Space Research. North-Holland Publishing Company. Amsterdam, Holland. (ACTIVE).

Life Support and Biosphere Science. Cognizant Communication Corporation. Elmsford, NY, USA. (ACTIVE).

Luftfahrtmedizin. 1936-1944. Springer. Berlin, Germany. (INACTIVE).

Luftfahrtmedizinische Abhandlungen. 1936-1939. G. Thieme. Leipzig, Germany. (INACTIVE).

Meddelanden Fran Flyg-Och Navalmedicinska Naemden. 1952-1963. Stockholm, Sweden. (INACTIVE).

La Médecine Aéronautique: Bulletin Du Service De Santé de L'Air. 1946-1959. L'Expansion Scientifique Francaise. Paris, France. (INACTIVE).

Médecine Aéronautique et Spatiale. Régies Édition Publicité. Paris, France. (ACTIVE).

Médecine Aéronautique et Spatiale - Médecine Subaquatique et Hyperbare. 1976-198u. Societe Francaise de Physiologie et De Médicine Aeronautiques et Cosmonautiques, Societe Francaise de Médicine Subaquatique et Hyperbare. Paris, France. (INACTIVE).

Medical Service Digest. Office of the Surgeon General, U.S. Air Force. Washington, D.C., USA. (ACTIVE).

Medicina Aeroespacial y Ambiental. Sociedad Española de Medicina Aeroespacial. (ACTIVE).

Mediko-Biologicheskie I Sotsial'no-Psikhologicheskie Problemy Osvoeniia Kosmosa I Regionov Zemli s Ekstremail'nymi Usloviiami Sushchestvovaniia. Institut Mediko-Biologicheskikh Problem. Moskva, Russia. (ACTIVE).

Military Medicine. Association of Military Surgeons of the United States. Bethesda, MD, USA. (ACTIVE).

Minerva Aerospaziale. Minerva Medica. Torino, Italy. (ACTIVE).

NASA Space Life Sciences Newsletter. Life and Biomedical Sciences and Applications Division. Washington, D.C., USA. (ACTIVE).

Nuevas del Aire. Cooperativa Española de Auxiliares de Vuelo de Aviación. Madrid, Spain. (ACTIVE).

Osterreichische Flugmedizinische Mitteilungen. Osterreichisches Institut fur Flugmedizin und Weltraumbiologie. Wien, Austria. (ACTIVE).

Proceedings of the Human Factors Society Annual Meeting. 1972-1992. Human Factors Society. Santa Monica, CA, USA. (INACTIVE).

Proceedings of the Human Factors and Ergonomics Society Annual Meeting. Human Factors and Ergonomics Society. Santa Monica, CA, USA (ACTIVE).

Publications of the School of Aerospace Medicine. School of Aerospace Medicine, U.S. Air Force. Brooks Air Force Base, Texas, USA. (ACTIVE).

Revista de Aeronáutica y Astronáutica. Ministerio de Defensa. Madrid, Spain. (ACTIVE).

Revista Médica da Aeronáutica. 1949-1970. Directoria de Saude da Aeronáutica. Rio de Janeiro, Brazil. (INACTIVE).

Revista Médica da Aeronáutica do Brasil. Diretoria de Saude da Força Aérea Brasileira. Rio de Janeiro, Brazil (ACTIVE).

Revista Sanidad de las Fuerzas Armadad de España. Hospital Militar Gomez Ulla. Madrid, Spain. (ACTIVE).

Revue de Médecine Aeronautique. 1961-1964. Societé Française de Physiologie et De Médicine Aeronautiques et Cosmonautiques, Societé Française de Médicine Subaquatique et Hyperbare. Paris, France. (INACTIVE).

Revue de Médecine Aeronautique et Spatiale. 1965-1975. Societé Francaise de Physiologie et De Médicine Aeronautiques et Cosmonautiques, Societé Francaise de Médicine Subaquatique et Hyperbare. Paris, France. (INACTIVE).

Revue des Corps de Santé des Armees: Terre, Mer, Air. 1960-1972. Centre de Recherches du Service de Santé des Armees. Paris, France. (INACTIVE).

Revue Internationale des Services de Santé des Armees de Terre, de Mer, et de L'Air. Office International de Documentation de Medicine Militaire. Paris, France. (ACTIVE).

Rivista di Medicina Aeronautica. 1938-1958. Associazione Culturale Aeronautica. (INACTIVE).

Rivista di Medicina Aeronautica e Spaziale. Editoriale Aeronautica. Rome, Italy. (ACTIVE).

Royal Thai Air Force Medical Gazette. 1952-1961. Bangkok, Thailand. (INACTIVE).

Safety On Line. U.S. Airways. Pittsburgh, PA, USA. (ACTIVE).

Section V. Journals, Newsletters, and Bulletins in Aerospace Medicine and Aerospace Human Factors

Sanidad Aeronáutica. Dirección General de Sanidad – Ministerio de Aeronáutica. Buenos Aires, Argentina. (ACTIVE).
Skysafety21: Korean Air Safety Magazine. Seoul, Korea. (ACTIVE).
The Society of U.S. Naval Flight Surgeons Newsletter. The Society of U.S. Naval Flight Surgeons. Naval Air Station Pensacola, FL, USA. (ACTIVE).
Space Biology and Aerospace Medicine. 1974-1979. Joint Publications Research Service. Arlington, VA, USA. (INACTIVE).
Space Bulletin. Gordon and Breach Science Publishers. Yverdon, Switzerland. (ACTIVE).
Space Energy and Transportation. 1996-2000. Sunsat Energy Council. Arlington, VA, USA. (INACTIVE).
Space Exploration. United States Superintendent of Documents. Washington, DC, USA. (ACTIVE).
Space Medicine Research Publications. National Aeronautics and Space Admininstration. Washington, D.C., USA. (ACTIVE).
Space Life Sciences. 1968-1973. Reidel Publishing Company. Dordrecht, Holland. (INACTIVE).
Studies in Aviation Medicine. 1943-1946. Yale University School of Medicine. New Haven, CT, USA. (INACTIVE).
Uchu Koku Kankyo Igaku. Nihon Uchu Kuku Kankyo Igakkai. Tokyo, Japan. (ACTIVE).
Undersea & Hyperbaric Medicine. Undersea and Hyperbaric Medical Society. Bethesda, MD, USA. (ACTIVE).
U.S. Air Force Medical Service Digest. 1950-1957. Office of the Surgeon General. Washington, DC, USA. (INACTIVE).
U.S. Army Aviation Digest. U.S. Army School of Aviation Medicine. Fort Rucker, Al, USA. (ACTIVE).
USSR Space Life Sciences Digest. National Aeronautics and Space Administration. Washington, D.C., USA. (ACTIVE).
Zentralblatt Fur Verkehrs-Medizin, Verkehrs-Psychologie, Luft-and Raumfahrt-Medizin. 1964-1973. Gesellschaft Fur Luft - Und Raumfahrt-Medizin, Deutsche Gesellschaft Fur Verkehrsmedizin. Munchen, Deutsche. (INACTIVE).

VI) ONLINE DATABASES CONTAINING BIBLIOGRAPHIC AND REGULATORY INFORMATION IN AEROSPACE MEDICINE AND RELATED DISCIPLINES

Aerospace Database (USA)
BIOSIS (USA)
CISTI (Canada – Internet)
Conference Papers Index (USA)
Current Contents Search (USA)
DTIC STINET (USA – Internet)
Embase:Exerpta Medica (The Netherlands)
ESA (European Space Agency)
FAA Incident Data System (USA – Internet)
Federal Aviation Regulations (USA – Internet)
ICYT (Spain)
IME (Spain)
Infotrack: Expanded Academic (USA – Internet)
INGENTA (United Kingdom – Internet)
Inside Conferences (United Kingdom)
Inside The British Library (United Kingdom – Internet)
JICST-EPLUS (Japan)
Joint Aviation Requirements (The Netherlands – Internet)
LC Marc – Books (USA)
MEDLINE (USA)
NASA Center For Aerospace Information: Reconplus (USA – Internet)
NASA Technical Reports Server (USA – Internet)
NTIS (USA - Internet)
NTSB Aviation Accident/Incident Database (USA – Internet)
OCLC Firstsearch (USA - Internet)
PASCAL (France)
PSYCINFO (USA)
PUBMED (USA – Internet)
REMARC (USA)
SCISEARCH (USA)
Spaceline (USA – Internet)
UK MARC (United Kingdom)

www.ingramcontent.com/pod-product-compliance
Lightning Source LLC
Chambersburg PA
CBHW081909170526
45167CB00007B/3208